CONSUMERS' GUIDE TO

Health Plans

BY THE EDITORS OF CONSUMERS' CHECKBOOK MAGAZINE

DISCARD

Consumers' CHECKBOOK is a program of the Center for the Study of Services, a nonprofit organization dedicated to helping consumers get the most for their money when they buy services. Founded in 1974, the Center is supported by subscribers to the two magazines it publishes in the Washington, DC, and San Francisco Bay areas, by sales of special books and reports in print and on the Web, by sales of other consumer information services, and by sales of survey, research, and analysis services. Its magazines, entitled *Washington Consumers' CHECKBOOK* and *Bay Area Consumers' CHECKBOOK*, rate the quality and prices of local service firms of various kinds, ranging from auto repair shops to banks to hospitals. The Center plans to begin publishing additional versions of *Consumers' CHECKBOOK* magazine in other metropolitan areas in the near future. This book is a special *Consumers' CHECKBOOK* publication.

The Center does survey, research, and analysis activities under contract with government agencies, employer coalitions, nonprofit public service organizations, and health plans, including many of the health plans reported on in this book, and receives financial compensation for this work from these organizations.

Consumers' CHECKBOOK
733 15th Street NW, Suite 820
Washington, DC 20005
202-347-7283
www.checkbook.org

Contents

Introduction

This book is intended to help you choose the health plan that is best for you. It will also help you deal with whatever plan you choose so that you get the best possible medical care and service. In Chapter 4, we give you plan-by-plan ratings, based on several sources.

A key source of information is an extensive survey in which ratings of individual plans were gathered from roughly 20,000 physicians who are currently, or were until recently, affiliated with the plans they rated. These physicians, many of whom have insider knowledge and perspective on what really goes on behind the scenes in plans they deal with, were asked to evaluate the aspects of plan performance that are important to consumers. In many cases, they gave strikingly higher ratings to some plans than to others.

Another source of information is a member satisfaction survey, in which members of all the rated plans were surveyed using the same basic questionnaire. The surveys were carried out by independent survey organizations, not by the plans themselves. In most cases, the surveys were carried out under extensive and tightly designed quality control procedures set up by the nonprofit National Committee for Quality Assurance (NCQA). We believe member survey data in this book cover more plans than have ever been rated this way in one publication before.

In addition, we have reported which plans distinguished themselves on a set of tightly defined measures of clinical performance—whether immunizations are given to the members who should have them, whether proper disease screening procedures are followed, whether proper medications are given in specific circumstances. And we have also reported plans' accreditation status with NCQA, which is the leading health plan accreditation agency.

You may, of course, wish to choose among plans we have not rated, including many traditional insurance plans. This book advises you on what to look for in any plan. We give special attention to the plan choices available to Medicare recipients and to your rights and benefits within the Medicare program.

Whichever plan you choose, you will need to deal with the plan effectively to assure that you get the care you deserve. We advise you on how to do that.

Top-Rated Plans

The plans listed here are those that received *Consumers' CHECKBOOK*'s top rating for quality. These plans were selected based on a scoring system *CHECKBOOK* has devised for this purpose. The scoring is based entirely on the data presented in the Plan Ratings table beginning on page 22, so you are free to make different selections based on the same data. In cases where some types of data were not available for a plan, the plan may have suffered a disadvantage in *CHECKBOOK*'s scoring.

Aetna U.S. Healthcare (HMO) (Northern Delaware and southern New Jersey)

Aetna U.S. Healthcare (HMO) (Southeastern Pennsylvania)

Anthem Blue Cross and Blue Shield (Connecticut)

Anthem Blue Cross and Blue Shield (Maine)

Anthem Blue Cross and Blue Shield (New Hampshire)

Anthem Blue Cross and Blue Shield (Ohio)

Arnett Health Plans (North-central Indiana)

AultCare (HMO) (Canton, OH area)

Blue Plus (Minnesota)

BlueCHiP (Southeastern Massachusetts and Rhode Island)

BlueCross BlueShield of Kansas City/ Blue-Care (HMO) (Kansas City area)

BlueCross BlueShield of Massachusetts/HMO Blue (MA, southeastern NH, and RI)

BlueCross BlueShield of North Carolina/Personal Care (North Carolina)

BlueCross BlueShield of Western New York/Community Blue (Western NY)

Bluegrass Family Health (Kentucky)

Capital District Physicians' Health Plan (Eastern Upstate New York)

Capital Health Plan (HMO) (Tallahassee, FL area)

Care Choices (HMO) (Central Michigan)

Carolina Care Plan (South Carolina)

CIGNA HealthCare of New Hampshire (New Hampshire)

CIGNA HealthCare of St. Louis (St. Louis area)

Companion HealthCare (South Carolina)

ConnectiCare (CT and southwestern MA)

Dean Health Plan (HMO) (Southern Wisconsin)

Empire BlueCross BlueShield (HMO) (Eastern and Downstate New York)

Excellus Health Plan/Blue Choice (Rochester, NY area)

First Priority Health (Northeastern Pennsylvania)

Florida Health Care Plans (Flagler and Volusia counties)

Geisinger Health Plan (Central and northeastern Pennsylvania)

Grand Valley Health Plan (HMO) (Grand Rapids, MI area)

Group Health Cooperative (HMO) (Northern Idaho and Washington)

Group Health Cooperative of Eau Claire (HMO) (Eau Claire, WI area)

Group Health Cooperative of South Central Wisconsin (HMO) (Madison, WI area)

Gunderson Lutheran Health Plan (HMO) (Southwestern Wisconsin)

HAP (HMO) (Southeastern Michigan and northwestern Ohio)

Harvard Pilgrim Health Care (Massachusetts and Maine)

Harvard Pilgrim Health Care of New England (New Hampshire and southern and eastern Vermont)

Health Alliance (Eastern Iowa and central and southern Illinois)

Health New England (Northern Connecticut and western Massachusetts)

Health Plan Hawaii (HMO) (Hawaii)

The Health Plan of the Upper Ohio Valley (HMO) (Parts of OH and WV)

HealthAmerica (HMO) (Parts of Ohio, Pennsylvania, and West Virginia)

HealthGuard (Harrisburg, Lancaster, Reading, and York areas)

HealthLink (HMO) (Parts of Arkansas, Illinois, and Missouri)

HealthPartners Classic (Twin Cities area)

HealthPlus of Michigan (Central MI)

HMO-CNY (HMO) (Central New York)

HMSA (Hawaii)

Independent Health (HMO) (Western NY)

John Deere Health Plan (HMO) (Parts of Iowa, Illinois, Tennessee, and Virginia)

Kaiser Permanente California (HMO) (Northern California)

Kaiser Permanente California (HMO) (Southern California)

Kaiser Permanente (Denver and Colorado Springs areas)

Kaiser Permanente Hawaii (HMO) (Hawaii)

Kaiser Permanente Northwest (HMO) (Corvallis, Portland, and Salem areas and southwestern Washington)

Keystone Health Plan Central (HMO) (Central Pennsylvania)

Keystone Health Plan West (Western Pennsylvania)

KPS Health Plans (HMO) (Puget Sound area)

M-CARE (HMO) (Southeastern Michigan)

Medica (Minnesota and western Wisconsin)

MVP Health Care (HMO) (Central and Eastern Upstate New York and the Southern Tier)

MVP Health Care (HMO) (Vermont)

NewAlliance Health Plan (Northwestern Pennsylvania)

Optima Health Plan (HMO) (Southeastern Virginia)

Optima Health Plan (POS) (Southeastern Virginia)

Oxford Health Plans (New York City, Long Island, and Downstate New York)

Paramount Health Care (HMO) (Southeastern Michigan and northwestern Ohio)

PersonalCare (HMO) (East-central Illinois)

Physicians Health Plan of Mid-Michigan (Central Michigan)

Preferred Care (Rochester, NY area)

Premera Blue Cross (Washington)

Premier Plus by Mercy Health Plans (HMO) (West-central Illinois and eastern Missouri)

Priority Health (HMO) (Most of western Michigan)

Providence Health Plans (Corvallis, Eugene, Portland, and Salem areas and southwestern Washington)

Rocky Mountain HMO (Colorado)

Scott & White Health Plan (HMO) (Austin and Waco areas)

Security Health Plan (HMO) (Northern, western, and central Wisconsin)

SummaCare (Northeastern Ohio)

Touchpoint Health Plan (HMO) (Northeastern Wisconsin)

Triple-S (HMO) (Puerto Rico)

Tufts Health Plan (HMO) (Massachusetts, southern New Hampshire, and Rhode Island)

Tufts Health Plan (POS) (Massachusetts, southern New Hampshire, and Rhode Island)

UnitedHealthcare of Florida (Florida)

UnitedHealthcare of New England (Southeastern and central Massachusetts and Rhode Island)

UnitedHealthcare of North Carolina (North Carolina)

UnitedHealthcare of Ohio (Dearborn County, IN, northern Kentucky, and southwestern Ohio)

UnitedHealthcare of Ohio (Central and southeastern Ohio)

UnitedHealthcare of Tennessee (Tennessee)

UnitedHealthcare of Texas (Austin, San Antonio, and Waco areas)

UnitedHealthcare of the Midlands (Western Iowa and eastern Nebraska)

UnitedHealthcare of the Midwest (Southern Illinois and most of eastern Missouri)

UnitedHealthcare of the Midwest (Eastern Kansas and most of western Missouri)

UnitedHealthcare of Wisconsin (Southeastern Wisconsin)

Univera Healthcare Western New York (Western New York)

UPMC Health Plan (Western PA)

Valley Health Plan (Western Wisconsin)

Chapter 1

Does It Matter Which Plan You Choose?

Which health plan you choose can have important consequences for the quality of health care you get, the convenience of getting that care, the ease and pleasantness of dealing with the plan, and your total health care costs. As background for this book, it is useful to have a little perspective on the nature of the plan-to-plan differences.

Quality Improvement Programs

Many health maintenance organizations (HMOs) make significant efforts—by working through doctors and by working with patients directly—to improve the quality of care their members receive.

There are many examples of quality improvement efforts—in which HMOs deliver substantially better care than patients could expect to receive from independent providers operating under a traditional insurance system. For example—

- Many plans have developed concerted programs to combat asthma— a leading cause of hospitalization, emergency room visits, and missed school days among children. These plans have—
  - ➡ Assembled experts to develop practice guidelines;
  - ➡ Distributed the guidelines broadly to practitioners;
  - ➡ Distributed educational materials to families with children having a history of asthma, explaining self-management techniques, how to keep a patient diary, how to use a peak flow meter to monitor changes in asthma symptoms, allergies that trigger asthma, and other information;
  - ➡ Distributed peak flow meters to help patients detect the onset of possible asthma attacks early;
  - ➡ Surveyed patients to find out about their health status and whether doctors were following practice guidelines;
  - ➡ Measured results like reductions in hospital admissions and increased use of appropriate anti-inflammatory medication— and reported progress on these measures back to physicians.
- Many plans have quality improvement programs to reduce coronary artery disease, the number one killer of both men and women in the U.S. One such plan focused on identifying members with cardiac disease, increasing the percentage of these members who were screened annually for LDL cholesterol, and increasing the percentage of screened members who had LDL levels below 130 mg/dL. The plan—
  - ➡ Developed lists of "at-risk" members, with the date of their last LDL measurement, and distributed the lists to medical groups so that the medical groups could reach out even to members who had not recently used medical group services;
  - ➡ Created financial incentives for medical groups to achieve superior performance on the LDL measures;
  - ➡ Developed telephone-based member-education services, including patient risk assessments and preparation of customized self-care plans;

- ➡ Offered a class with one-on-one counseling for at-risk members;
- ➡ Offered basic and advanced cholesterol classes and a program that included instruction on a very low-fat, plant-based diet;
- ➡ Distributed bulletins to medical groups on the appropriate use of statin drugs to help control LDL levels;
- ➡ Authorized practitioners to write prescriptions for health education classes at local community colleges;
- ➡ Implemented a "Better Health Restaurant Challenge" to increase the availability of low-fat foods in local restaurants, with registered dieticians evaluating menu items and a contest for the best tasting, low-fat items;
- ➡ Hired a plan staff member to coordinate many of these activities.

You will want to look for plans that carry on such quality improvement programs. The information on individual plans evaluated in this book will give you indications of which plans have been successfully running such programs.

Delays and Denials

Quality improvement programs are the upside of what health plans can contribute to your medical care; the most troublesome downside is the possibility that plans will inappropriately deny or delay care. Such denials and delays have made health plans the frequent brunt of jokes and have made HMO-bashing a sure source of applause lines in movies and public speeches. Widely reported cases include—

- **The case of Mrs. R.** Mrs. R enrolled in a large HMO. She began having bladder discomfort and went to her primary care physician. The doctor referred her to a urologist, but the first available appointment was nearly three weeks away. In the meantime, Mrs. R began bleeding from her urinary tract. She went to the emergency room. The ER doctors wanted to admit her to the hospital and called for authorization from the HMO. Authorization was denied. Mrs. R went home. She returned to the ER the following day, bleeding even more heavily. Again, the ER doctors requested authorization to admit her. Again, it was denied. Mrs. R went home. The following day, when Mrs. R went to the emergency room, she was bleeding so heavily that she had to walk with bath towels between her legs. Again the HMO refused authorization to admit her to the hospital. Finally, in desperation, Mrs. R's son took her to another hospital. The doctors there discovered a tumor the size of a grapefruit in Mrs. R's bladder, admitted her on an emergency basis and rushed her to surgery. Because of the loss of blood over the preceding days, Mrs. R suffered a heart attack during the surgery. Although she survived, her health was seriously compromised.
- **The case of Mr. L.** Mr. L was diagnosed with lung cancer. His plan oncologist told him that the tumor was too close to his heart and that he could, therefore, only be treated with radiation therapy. After the

health plan refused Mr. L's request for an outside consultation with a surgical oncologist and because the plan did not have a surgical oncologist available, Mr. L paid for on his own a consultation with a university-affiliated specialist. That specialist told Mr. L that the tumor was, in fact, operable, although it would be a very delicate and tricky operation. The surgeon also told Mr. L that the surgery was his only chance for survival because radiation therapy simply could not eradicate the tumor and, in addition, was likely to damage his heart. Even more frightening, the surgeon also informed Mr. L that the tumor was growing very fast and could double in size within 30 days. As such, it was imperative that the surgery occur as soon as possible. Mr. L then had to start the referral and review process within the HMO to get approval. He had to go back to his primary care physician for a referral to the in-plan oncologist and then had to go to a consultation with the in-plan oncologist. The in-plan oncologist concurred that surgery was the best possible treatment and that it had to be done immediately, but that the plan had no surgeons qualified to perform the surgery. Thus, the oncologist recommended, the plan should authorize out-of-plan treatment. The plan denied the treatment. That process, alone, took one week. Mr. L simply did not have the luxury of waiting for the plan's internal grievance process to review the issue and he certainly did not have the time to have an external review process deal with the issue. He had to have the surgery immediately. He disenrolled from the health plan the next day and the day after that had the surgery—which was paid for by Medicare. He is still alive and well, four years later.

Problems like these are clearly not the norm in HMOs. But they are not as rare as one would hope—especially in light of the fact that, in any given year, most members don't have medical conditions that put their plans to the test. Results from a survey of members of 268 plans in 2001 reveal that, on average, four percent reported having "a big problem" getting the care the member or a doctor believed was necessary and nine percent reported having "a big problem" getting a referral to a specialist that the member needed to see. In 23 of the plans, more than eight percent of members reported having "a big problem" getting the care the member or a doctor believed was necessary, and in 21 of the plans, more than 15 percent reported having "a big problem" getting a referral to a specialist that the member needed to see. The information in this book on individual plans will give you some indication of the plans in which you are at greatest risk of having such experiences.

Choice of Doctors and Help Choosing

Any HMO that creates financial hurdles to your seeing any doctor of your choice might have a negative effect on the care you could otherwise arrange. This can be a serious problem if a plan offers a limited list of doctors or a list that does not include the best doctors.

But many HMOs offer a vast selection of physician choices. In addition, an HMO can assist you by screening out the most incompetent doctors; HMO accreditation standards (although not always successfully carried out) require plans to check the credentials of physicians to be sure that at least they are medical school graduates and have not been barred from practice by state disciplinary boards. And some HMOs provide information to help members select good doctors. A number of plans list information on training and credentials in their provider directories, and a few even include information on how surveyed patients have rated each doctor and how the doctor has scored on a few measures of clinical care. You will want to look hard at the information each plan provides you about its participating doctors, and you will want to look at the plan's provider lists to see if the doctors and hospitals offered include ones you

would want to use—especially doctors you are already using.

You will find substantial differences. For example, when a list of the highest rated doctors in another *Consumers' CHECKBOOK* publication, our *Guide to Top Doctors*, was matched against the provider lists of four HMOs in a major metropolitan area, one plan offered 59 percent of these top doctors, two offered between 40 and 45 percent, and one offered only 27 percent. Such differences could have significant consequences for the quality of care you are likely to get.

The plan-by-plan information in this book will give you extensive information on the quality of doctors members can expect to see in each plan. You will see how the doctors are rated by members, by other physicians, and on direct measures of the care they provide.

Convenience and Service

You will also be interested in the convenience and ease of getting care from different plans. Some plans will allow you to self-refer to specialists, but others require you to go through a primary care doctor for every referral. Most HMOs spare you the bother of having to do much claims paperwork, but paperwork can be extensive with traditional insurance plans. Most plans give you a wide choice of doctors' office locations, but a few require you to choose among a limited number of clinics. You will want to check for yourself how plans you are considering are organized, where you have to go for care, what the referral rules are, and how you will pay. In this book, you will find information on each plan's claims handling processes and paperwork hassles and on the level of service members report getting from customer service staff.

The plan-by-plan comparisons in this book will also give you information on the convenience of dealing with physicians' offices. You'll find information on how long members typically wait for appointments, how long members spend waiting in doctors' offices, and how easy it is to get advice by phone from doctors' offices. These are measures that depend more on the doctor than on anything the plan can do. But some plans may be more successful than others in recruiting doctors who are sensitive to members' needs and in prodding doctors to provide convenient service.

Costs

Depending on which plan you join, you might have thousands of dollars more or less per year in health care costs. The costs to you are not only your share of premiums but also out-of-pocket costs for deductibles, copayments, and items the plan doesn't cover.

It is not possible in a book like this to compare what each plan will cost each reader—although we have provided a relative-cost index for many of the plans in the plan-by-plan ratings in Chapter 4. Your actual premiums and out-of-pocket costs will depend on your age, family size, health condition, where you live, and other factors. In addition, what you pay will depend on the specific premium and benefit package that you buy as an individual or that your employer purchases from a plan. If you get insurance through your employment, what you pay will also depend on how much your employer contributes to the cost.

If you have plan choices, you will need to look carefully at the costs of each option. This is particularly important if one of your choices is a traditional fee-for-service plan, since out-of-pocket costs play a bigger role in such plans. In Chapter 5, you will find a worksheet to help you compare costs.

Why Plan-to-Plan Differences Are Smaller Than They Might Have Been

Although there are important differences among plans, the differences are not as dramatic as might have been expected 30 years ago when the

HMO movement was first starting on a period of major expansion. At that time, most of the HMOs were facilities-based plans: each had its own limited group of doctors, those doctors worked for only one plan, and care was delivered in the plan's own clinics. These HMOs had the potential to exercise powerful control over medical policies and practices, over management and information systems, and over the environment in which care was delivered. One could anticipate that, as these plans evolved, each plan's participating doctors would begin to adhere to similar practice guidelines, and that there would be tight coordination among all the participating practitioners. One could imagine that the plans that used their control to educate and inform doctors, measure performance, and push toward the most up-to-date, well-managed care would prosper in the marketplace as the quality of their care was recognized by the employers, consumers, and public agencies who would be purchasing plan services.

As the health care system has evolved, however, plans' control of care, and therefore the importance of plan choice, has turned out not to be as great as might have been expected. The system has evolved on a different path.

In the early years of HMO expansion, beginning in the early 1970s, most plans strove to distinguish themselves by cutting costs rather than focusing on managing for superior quality. They took this cost-cutting path in part because it was relatively easy to do and in part because that is where they were getting pressure from purchasers of their services, who could judge costs more easily than quality.

An easy way to cut costs was to cut the amount of costly care given. It was well known that much care in hospitals—the number of admissions, the length of each stay, and the medical care services given during each stay—was wasteful. Much care was not helpful—in fact, was possibly harmful—to patients' health. Even many tests and treatments given in doctors' offices were of doubtful value—possibly resulting from the financial incentives doctors had under the traditional fee-for-service system, which gave the doctor more income if he or she provided more service.

HMOs went about their cutting of costs—and services—in various ways—

- More and more health plans began paying hospitals based on the type of case—the disease to be treated or surgery to be performed—rather than the number of days, tests, treatments, and other services provided. So hospitals had an incentive to cut services.
- Most HMOs required each patient to choose a primary care physician who would serve as a gatekeeper, with the patient required to get approval and a referral from this physician before getting care from specialists, hospitals, or other providers.
- Some HMOs paid doctors or medical groups based on the number of patients the doctor or group was responsible for (referred to as capitation payment) rather than the services provided. So more services meant more work and cost for the doctor for the same income.
- Some HMOs paid doctors and medical groups bonuses for keeping down the number of services provided, the number of referrals to specialists, and the number of hospitalizations. Some actually docked practitioners' pay for using or prescribing what the plan regarded as too many services.
- Most HMOs—and also other less restrictive plans like preferred provider organizations (PPOs) and even traditional insurance plans—began to require approval from plan administrators before many types of surgery, hospitalization, or other specialty care.

HMOs' cost cutting was good for the nation's cost of living—and probably also for the quality of health care, by sparing patients much unnecessary, unpleasant, and often dangerous care. And it wasn't all done by asserting control over care providers. It was also done by documenting the appropriateness of lower-cost types of care—by educating doctors and other providers, and consumers.

But cutting services obviously has the potential to go too far, and even a system that generally makes appropriate cuts can sometimes make mistakes. As HMO enrollment increased, consumers and the employers who purchase plan services for most consumers worried that HMOs with tight controls over care might deny needed care. More loosely configured plans appeared to some to be less of a threat to good care. Many consumers and employers preferred the sense of greater control they would have in a plan that allowed them a wide choice of providers.

In addition, many consumers balked at the idea of giving up their current physicians to join a plan that offered access to only a limited number of physicians. And many did not like the idea of having to go for their care to a plan clinic that might be inconvenient and bureaucratic. Companies selecting plans for their employees often favored plans that had the largest panels of participating doctors so that few employees would have to give up their existing relationships with their doctors.

What's more, many doctors wanted to practice in the same kind of solo or small group setting that they had become accustomed to. They had no interest in joining up with a plan that would require them to work in a large clinic environment.

Faced with all these forces, most HMOs did not expand in the model of the early forerunners. Instead, most HMOs grew as loosely configured panels of doctors who worked in individual or group practice settings and simply contracted with plans. Each of these loosely configured HMOs has many more doctors than it would need to care for its own members, and each physician or group is generally affiliated with a number of HMOs.

In recent years, in fact, the health plan market has continued to evolve toward even looser structures. Many plans now offer a point of service (POS) option that lets members use any specialist of their choice without referral from a primary care physician—so long as the patient agrees to pay a higher co-payment than would be required if the member got a referral by a plan primary care physician to a plan-affiliated specialist. More and more HMOs allow members to self-refer to affiliated specialists—to skip the process of getting a referral from a gatekeeper primary care physician. And PPOs, which don't even include a gatekeeper referral system, have recently been expanding more rapidly than HMOs.

The loose structure of these plans means their control is limited—for better or worse.

The good side of limited control, from the patient's standpoint, is that the HMO must be careful not to be too restrictive in the care and services it allows. If it is too restrictive, it risks losing both patients and doctors. The doctors can cut their affiliations and simply work for the HMO's competitors or serve more non-HMO patients. Such dis-affiliation will affect only a fraction of the doctor's patients—and even some of them might be able to come back to the doctor by switching to another HMO or to another type of plan that offers greater flexibility.

On the other hand, the lack of tight control exercised by loosely structured HMOs means that no plan has very strong incentives to push its doctors to the highest level of care quality. For example—

- If an HMO offers fabulous education programs for its doctors, its competitors, for whom the doctors also work, may benefit almost as much as it does.
- If the HMO invests heavily in developing practice guidelines to assist doctors in making the best possible medical decisions, its competitors benefit.
- If the HMO invests in the most important area for potential advancement of modern medical care—the development of computerized

medical record systems that let doctors efficiently share information, follow patient progress, and get helpful diagnosis and treatment suggestions at the time of each medical decision—the HMO's competitors benefit from the fact that the doctors equipped and trained to use these systems will use the systems for the competitors' members as well.

The fact that the health plan marketplace has not evolved into the system of all-powerful and sharply distinct competing HMOs means that HMOs are not the dominant players in the health care system they might have been, and your choice of plan is not as critical as it might have been. But choosing a good plan is still very important, and this book should help you.

Chapter 2

What Choices Do You Have?

You may have a wide range of health plan choices open to you, or your choices may be more limited. But very likely you can have at least some influence in decisions about your health care coverage.

Most Americans have health insurance coverage through their employers. Some employers offer a single plan. Others offer a number of choices. Choice is good for consumers. It allows you the opportunity to choose a plan that best fits your needs, and it makes plans compete for your enrollment. Such competition, just like competition among car manufacturers, restaurants, or any other type of business, can create incentives for continuing improvement in quality and efficiency.

If you work for a large employer that offers more than one plan, ask the employer for as much information as it can give you on each plan. You can then use this book to assist you in putting together more information to help you choose the plan that's best for you.

If your employer offers only one plan or a limited selection of plans, you can compare what you're offered to the range of other plans available in your community. If the other plans seem like they would be better choices for you and some other employees, you might ask your employer to add one or more plans to its offerings. Some plans require small employers—for example, employers with fewer than 20 employees—to contract exclusively with a single plan. But it is generally easy for larger employers to offer several plan choices.

If you work for a small employer that will only offer a single plan, you can volunteer to do research on available plans to help the employer choose the one that is the best choice for the most employees.

Unfortunately, many Americans have no health insurance coverage. That's a very uncomfortable situation. A serious health problem can be staggeringly expensive. Treatment of heart disease with bypass surgery, for instance, is likely to cost more than $40,000. Even a three-day stay in a hospital generally costs more than $4,000.

If you have no health insurance coverage, this book might give you some assistance by helping you find the most affordable plans that provide adequate coverage and high-quality care.

If you are employed (including self-employed), your best approach for getting health plan coverage is to do it through your employer. You can give this book to your employer or offer to do the work of finding a good plan for your employer. There are substantial advantages to buying health plan coverage through an employment-related group.

First, some health plans offer coverage at lower rates to employed groups than to individuals. The plans offer these better rates because they believe employed persons are less likely to be sick than are persons who aren't working. Also, they know that by insuring a group they can expect to get some healthy individuals, not just unhealthy individuals who particularly want insurance. In addition, they allow for the fact that dealing with a group rather than individuals reduces administrative costs.

Second, there are substantial tax breaks for employment-related purchase of health insurance. The dollar amount of the premiums a company pays is deductible as a business expense by the employer, it is not subject to the employer share of payroll taxes, and it escapes both payroll taxes and income taxes for the employee.

Third, there is a broader selection of good plans available to employment-based groups than is available to individuals.

You'll want to push your employer to offer coverage. It even makes sense for you and other employees to consider giving up salary or wages in exchange for the employer's commitment to put an equivalent amount into health insurance premiums.

If you are unemployed or can't get your employer to purchase insurance, you still have many health insurance choices. Many plans sell coverage to individuals.

You can get help shopping for a plan from insurance agents and brokers listed in the Yellow Pages of your phone directory. Some agents can tell you about many different plans, but some sell only a single company's plans or have financial incentives to favor a particular company. If you want to get a good picture of your range of choices, you'll do well to talk with several agents. Some plans—including many HMOs—expect you to contract directly with them, not through an agent.

If you are a professional, you might also want to consider getting coverage through an association you're qualified to join. Compare the association's plan to what you can get on your own.

If you are eligible for Medicare, you have a large number of choices. There are insurance policies that simply fill in the gaps that Medicare doesn't cover; there are health maintenance organization plans that will take over complete responsibility for your care; and many employers offer plans that continue to cover employees or retirees who have become eligible for Medicare. The special options for persons eligible for Medicare are discussed in Chapter 6.

Low-income consumers on Medicaid also may have health plan choices. Many states now contract with health maintenance organizations to take over full responsibility for care of Medicaid recipients. Your state Medicaid agency can give you a list of plan options open to you.

Chapter 3

Types of Plans

Health plans today come in many forms. There are traditional indemnity insurance plans, health maintenance organizations (HMOs), preferred provider organizations (PPOs), point-of-service HMOs (POS HMOs), and other models.

Traditional Plans

With a traditional, indemnity plan, in exchange for your premium, the plan agrees to pay all or a share of the cost of services you use. There is typically a list of covered services, such as doctors' office visits and hospital stays, and a set of limitations or exclusions, such as an exclusion of coverage for cosmetic surgery. You can use virtually any licensed provider of the covered services—physicians, hospitals, etc.—and the plan pays the provider or reimburses you when you file claims for what you've paid the provider. You can decide for yourself when and where to get services.

Usually these plans have an annual "deductible"—an amount you must pay from your own pocket before the plan pays anything. In some plans, called "catastrophic plans," this deductible is set very high—say, $1,000 or $5,000—so that the plan steps in only when expenses are so high that they would be financially disastrous for you.

Usually you also have to pay "coinsurance" out of your own pocket. Coinsurance is a portion of each service charge—say, 20 percent of the charge for each doctor's office visit. Most indemnity plans have an annual "out-of-pocket limit" on the amount you will have to put out in coinsurance payments. After the limit is reached, the plan pays 100 percent of charges. But usually certain services—for example, psychiatric services—are excluded from the limit, and the limit doesn't apply to fees charged by doctors or other health care providers to the extent that those fees exceed fee maximums set by the plan.

Since doctors and other providers are paid on a "fee-for-service" basis (a fee for each office visit, test, procedure, or other service they deliver), a provider makes more money by prescribing and delivering more services.

These indemnity plans once dominated the market, but now—because they have less control of costs than other types of plans—are much less common.

HMOs

At the other extreme from indemnity insurance plans are HMOs. In the basic HMO plan model—

- You are expected to get all your care from a list of doctors, hospitals, and other providers affiliated with the plan.
- You are expected to select a primary care doctor—usually a general practitioner, family practitioner, internist, or (for children) pediatrician—to provide your basic care and to be the "gatekeeper" who refers you to other services. The plan won't pay for care by a

specialist, hospital, or other provider unless preapproved by the gatekeeper (except in an emergency).
- Participating physicians get no financial gain (and may even bear a share of the costs) if the quantity of services (days in hospital, office visits, etc.) their patients receive is deemed by the plan to be too high.
- The plan pays doctors, hospitals, and other participating providers without your having to file claims. Your out-of-pocket costs are minor—though you may have to pay providers modest "copayments" of, for example, $10 or $20 per office visit.

HMOs come in many forms. One model is a "facility-based" HMO, in which the doctors work in the plan's own clinics. These doctors are usually on salary and work only for one plan. Plans of this type are sometimes referred to as "group practice" plans or "staff model" plans.

Another model is an "individual practice association" (IPA) in which individual doctors contract with the plan but practice in their own private offices. Usually these doctors also see nonplan patients, and the same doctor may see patients from several different HMOs.

A third model is a "network" plan, sometimes referred to as a "mixed model" plan. The network plan contracts with IPAs and participating medical groups. A participating medical group is a group of physicians who work together in a group practice facility, or "multispecialty clinic." The IPAs and participating medical groups, in turn, contract with individual physicians. These physicians typically see non-HMO patients as well as HMO patients, and a participating medical group or IPA may contract with several different HMOs.

PPOs

A PPO health plan falls between an HMO and a traditional indemnity plan. A PPO typically has contracts with many individual physicians, hospitals, and other providers in the community. A provider may be a member of several different PPOs and several HMOs and may also serve many non-PPO, non-HMO patients. A PPO's providers agree to a discounted fee schedule for the PPO's patients. If you use a PPO provider, you pay the provider either a percentage (say, 10 percent) of the discounted fee or a fixed copayment (say, $10 per office visit). But you can also use any other provider who is not connected with the PPO if you are willing to pay more for the service.

If you go outside the list of PPO providers, you may pay extra for two reasons. First, a PPO has a schedule setting the highest fees it will pay non-PPO providers. If your doctor charges more than that fee schedule (say, $100 for an office visit rather than the $80 the PPO's fee schedule allows), you have to pay the difference ($20 in this example). Second, the percentage you must pay non-PPO providers is usually higher than the percentage you pay when using a PPO provider. For example, a PPO plan might require you to pay 30 percent of the PPO's allowable fee schedule amount when you use non-PPO doctors, compared to 10 percent of the discounted fee when using PPO doctors. In addition, some PPOs make you pay a deductible—say, the first $300 of your year's medical expenses—out of your own pocket when using a non-PPO provider but let you skip the deductible when you use PPO providers.

Although you pay extra to go outside a PPO's provider list, most PPOs, like most indemnity plans, have an annual upper limit on what they expect you to pay out of your own pocket. For example, a plan's rule may be that the plan will pay 100 percent of costs after you've paid $3,000 out of your own pocket. (This limit won't apply to provider charges that are above the plan's allowable fee schedule.)

So a PPO does give you more flexibility than an HMO to go to a world-renowned treatment center or just to use a particular doctor your brother-in-law thought was great.

Another important difference between PPOs and HMOs is that PPOs allow you to get specialist and hospital care without having to be referred by your "gatekeeper" primary care physician. As a PPO member, if you want to go directly to a dermatologist, orthopedic surgeon, psychiatrist, or other specialist, you can simply call the specialist and set up an appointment. If the specialist prescribes a procedure (perhaps a CAT scan), you can have it done without your primary care doctor's approval. If you don't like the results with one specialist, you can call another. (Even in PPOs and traditional indemnity plans, the doctor of your choice will have some decisions reviewed. Most plans require the doctor to get plan approval at least before doing surgery or putting you in the hospital.)

Other Types of Plans

There are many other variations in health plan models. One popular model is the point-of-service (POS) HMO. This model is an HMO combined with an indemnity insurance plan. If you select a primary care doctor from the HMO's list of doctors and use only that doctor and the providers that doctor refers you to, the plan functions just like any other HMO. But you also have the option of using any other physician and referring yourself to specialists and other nonparticipating providers just as you would in a traditional indemnity insurance plan. If you go outside of HMO procedures in this way, however, you will have deductibles and coinsurance requirements and you are responsible for charges above the plan's fee schedule, just as you would be if you were in an indemnity plan or if you went to nonparticipating providers in a PPO. Like PPOs and indemnity insurance plans, most POS HMOs have an annual limit on what you'll have to pay out of pocket. (As in those other types of plans, the limit does not apply to charges in excess of the plan's fee schedule.)

Another increasingly popular variant is an HMO without a gatekeeper. In a plan of that type, you are limited to the HMO's list of primary care doctors and specialists, but you can go to one of the plan's specialists without getting a referral from a primary care doctor.

Which Type of Plan Is Best?

Among the various plan types, basic HMOs are most restrictive. They limit your choice of providers and they limit you to getting only services that are approved by your primary care doctor. HMO plans without a gatekeeper give you a little more control of your care and a lot more convenience. POS HMO plans and PPO plans give you even more flexibility but are more restrictive than a traditional indemnity insurance plan if you want to keep your out-of-pocket expenses to a minimum.

So, why accept plan restrictions? One reason is cost. HMOs are generally less expensive than the other types of plans—lower premiums and lower out-of-pocket costs. POS HMOs and PPO plans also tend to be less

expensive than indemnity plans—but more expensive than HMOs. The cost differences among plan types are not always large, however, and the pattern is not consistent. In fact, some indemnity and PPO plans are actually less expensive than some HMOs (see table below).

Costs of Different Types of Plans
(Premiums plus estimated average out-of-pocket costs for single person)

	Lowest priced one-tenth of plans	Average plan	Highest priced one-tenth of plans
HMO and POS plans	$2880	$3555	$4230
PPO using PPO providers	$3760	$4620	$5090
PPO not using PPO providers	$3920	$4939	$5430

These are estimated 2002 costs (combined for employer and employee) for a sample of plans in the Federal Employees Health Benefits Program, as reported in Checkbook's 2002 Guide to Health Plans for Federal Employees.

Another reason to prefer an HMO would be if you believe it has better doctors on its list of providers than the average doctor in your community. By choosing an excellent HMO, you might increase your chances of being treated by high-quality doctors—compared to your chances if you must choose doctors for yourself under an indemnity plan. (A PPO plan also could include an unusually high proportion of quality providers on its list, though PPOs tend to be less selective than HMOs in their provider recruitment.) But comparison of HMO provider lists to the lists of highly recommended specialists in *CHECKBOOK's Guide to Top Doctors* indicates that in many communities the most highly regarded doctors tend to be affiliated with few (if any) HMOs. How good or bad a particular HMO's—or PPO's—doctors in fact are compared to other doctors in the community depends on the attractiveness of the compensation and working conditions the plan offers and the effectiveness of its recruiting, screening, and quality monitoring efforts.

HMOs might have another virtue—an ability to improve medical care quality in a way that indemnity plans and PPOs cannot—by guiding and supporting the way doctors, nurses, and other providers practice and by educating patients directly. A sports analogy may illustrate the point. Not only does an HMO have a relatively high degree of control over the team it recruits to deliver your medical care; it also has the opportunity to coach and support its players. It can try to get them to use new medical care techniques and better ways of communicating with patients. And it may be able to give them especially good facilities and equipment.

The coaching and management possibilities can be seen in the way some plans have improved the treatment of asthma and cardiovascular care, as described in Chapter 4. This kind of improvement in physician practice can be done most easily in a facility-based HMO. A facility-based plan usually has a relatively small number of physicians, and most work for this one plan full-time. The plan can collect information on what each doctor does, train those who need to change, and then follow up the results.

In contrast, a PPO or IPA-type HMO can't get as much information on what each doctor is doing in his or her private office. Also, training the hundreds of primary care physicians that participate in a typical PPO or IPA-type HMO is more difficult. In fact, no PPO or IPA-type plan has much incentive to train its doctors because the doctors also work for various other plans. Finally, a doctor might not respond to one plan's efforts to change the way he or she practices medicine if that plan provides only a small portion of the doctor's business.

Although lack of plan control limits a plan's ability to drive quality improvement, less control may be a virtue if a plan would not use the control to push for such improvement. Indeed, a plan with control could use its control to push doctors toward cutting back appropriate but costly types of care.

Given the possible advantages and disadvantages of different plan types, and different levels of restrictions and plan control, no plan type is a clear winner for all consumers. Some consumers will be more concerned than others about the restrictiveness of HMOs, and some may weigh HMOs' cost advantages or care management potential especially heavily. Even if you prefer one plan type in theory, you might choose a plan of another type because you believe that specific plan is extraordinary.

Chapter 4

Choosing a Plan: Finding Top-Quality Medical Care and Service

Choosing a health plan that gives high-quality care and service might save your health or your life—and it will certainly make getting care more pleasant and convenient.

Although cost and breadth of coverage are important, for many consumers quality comes first. A 1995 survey of more than 50,000 Federal employees, using a questionnaire *Consumers' CHECKBOOK* developed, asked respondents to rank the health plan features most important to them personally. As the figure to the right shows, 45 percent said "quality of care" was most important, 16 percent gave greatest weight to "doctors available through plan (being able to find doctors you're satisfied with)," and 13 percent considered "access to care (ease of arranging for and getting care)" most important. That makes a total of 74 percent who gave greatest importance to one or another of these three aspects of care quality.

Although these aspects of quality matter to consumers, other research has indicated that many consumers focus on cost in selecting plans because they don't believe there are major quality differences among plans or don't believe the available data reveal which plans are better or worse in ways that matter to them.

If you are selecting among traditional indemnity plans, of course, there is relatively little room for plan-to-plan variation in medical care quality. All indemnity plans let you choose among virtually the entire pool of providers in the community and no plan has much influence over how the doctors and other providers practice medicine or deal with their patients. Some indemnity plans may be more restrictive in deciding whether to approve hospitalization, surgery, or certain other procedures, but for most patients these plan-to-plan differences are relatively small.

Among PPOs, there is more room for quality variation—because of differences in the lists of participating providers. Again, however, the plan-to-plan differences are relatively small.

Among HMOs, in contrast, quality differences can be significant. So most of the information in this chapter is focused on selecting among HMOs.

The Plan Ratings table, beginning on page 22, gives information to help guide you to a good plan. In Appendix A, you will find a description of the sources of this information. Beginning on page 20 is a discussion of important limitations and issues in the interpretation of some of the data, based on our extensive experience collecting and analyzing such data.

Can You Keep Your Current Doctor or Doctors?

Before considering the kinds of information on the Plan Ratings table, you can check one key point on your own for each plan: will you be able, after joining the plan, to continue using doctors with whom you currently have a good relationship?

Keeping current doctors spares you from wasting time and effort finding new doctors you like and with whom you can communicate easily. In addition, if you have had a good doctor for a period of time, that doctor will have the advantage of knowing you, understanding your medical history, and being able to communicate with you better than with a new patient.

By choosing an indemnity plan, you avoid the need to sever any doctor relationships. The same is true of PPO plans or point-of-service HMOs if you are willing to pay extra to use doctors who are not on the plan's provider list. But if you are considering HMOs or you want to keep costs to a minimum in a PPO or point-of-service HMO, you'll want to check where your doctors are affiliated. To find out about your doctors' affiliations, you can check plans' provider lists in print or on the Web. Or you can simply call your doctors' offices and ask. (Even if a physician is listed in a plan's provider directory, a call to the office is a good idea; over time, affiliations change.) If you, your spouse, and your children all have several doctors you use and like, you probably won't be able to find a new HMO that includes them all. You will have to decide which physician relationships are most important to you.

Here is a point to keep in mind: in a plan that contracts with physician groups rather than individual doctors, a particular specialist listed in the plan's provider directory might not be accessible to you easily, or at all, depending on the doctor you choose as your primary care physician. Your primary care physician's group might have rules, backed up by strong financial incentives, directing its physicians to refer only to specific specialists affiliated with the group. That might mean just a single allergist, a single rheumatologist, etc.

If you are considering a plan that contracts with a network of groups, be sure to think ahead to which primary care physician you will be using and how that might limit your choices of specialists, hospitals, and other providers. Ask the plan for a description of referral arrangements. Also, talk with one or more of the plan's primary care doctors and ask how much flexibility you would have in requesting a specific specialist: would you be able to choose to use any specialist affiliated with the plan or only one of the specialists affiliated with the doctor's own physician group?

Which Plans Look Best Overall?

Turning now to the information on the Plan Ratings table that begins on page 22, there are several kinds of measures that bear on the overall quality of a plan. A key overall indicator is the score each plan received from surveyed doctors when asked to rate the "overall quality of the HMO for patient care." Results are shown for doctors who said either that they were currently affiliated with the plan or that they had been affiliated with the plan in the past two years. These doctors have had a chance to observe programs and incentives plans may have set up to help doctors practice better medicine and to educate and inform members. They have also had the opportunity to see whether the plans have created obstacles to good care.

The Plan Ratings table shows the percentage of the doctors who rated the plan either "good," "very good," or "excellent." As you can see, there are striking plan-to-plan differences, with some plans getting such favorable ratings from more than 80 percent of the doctors who rated them and others getting such ratings from fewer than 30 percent.

Another key indicator of overall quality is ratings by members who were asked to rate "all of your experience with your health plan" on a zero to 10 scale, with zero representing the "worst health plan possible" and 10 representing the "best health plan possible." The Plan Ratings table shows the percent of surveyed members who rated each plan 8, 9, or 10. The Plan Ratings table also shows results on a member survey question that is focused somewhat more narrowly—on overall *health care* rather than the overall *plan*—using the same zero to 10 scale.

In addition, the Plan Ratings table includes another overall indicator of overall quality from the survey of members: the percentage of members who reported having called or written the plan in the previous 12 months with a complaint or problem. Unfortunately, the member survey question did not distinguish between complaints and problems, and some problems might not reflect badly on a plan. But to the extent that the question suggests the presence of complaints, you will want to favor plans that show low percentages on the Plan Ratings table.

A different type of overall quality indicator, also reported on the Plan Ratings table, is accreditation status. There are three organizations that accredit health plans: the National Committee for Quality Assurance (NCQA) accredits the largest number of plans; the Joint Commission on the Accreditation of Healthcare Organizations (JCAHO), which has long been the accrediting organization for hospitals, accredits a smaller number of plans (or "health care networks"); a third organization, the American Accreditation HealthCare Commission, accredits only a few plans, although it accredits a significant number of other types of health care organizations. Accreditation through all of these organizations is voluntary, although some large employers require it for plans that wish to serve their employees. Plans pay substantial fees to be accredited. The Plan Ratings table indicates whether plans were accredited as of a specific date in early 2002—and it indicates the level of accreditation each plan had achieved. (If a plan was accredited by both NCQA and one of the other organizations, only the NCQA accreditation is listed.)

Since NCQA accreditation is the most widespread type, it is most useful for comparing plans, and we focus on it here.

Accreditation by NCQA requires an extensive review by physicians and managed care experts both on-site and on paper. A portion of what goes into accreditation decisions is plan scores on the member surveys for which we have reported results in some detail on the Plan Ratings table. Plans' performance on direct measures of the clinical care doctors provide, highlights of which are also shown on the table, provide an additional input into the accreditation decision. But the reviewers also must make more subjective judgments based on plan documents and on observations and information gathered on site visits. NCQA describes its 60 accreditation standards as falling into the following five categories—

- **Access and Service.** Do health plan members have access to the care and service they need? For example, are doctors in the health plan free to discuss all treatment options available? Do patients report having problems getting needed care? How well does the health plan follow up on grievances?
- **Qualified Providers.** Does the health plan assess each doctor's qualifications and what members say about their providers? Does the health plan regularly check the licenses and training of physicians? How do health plan members rate their personal doctor or nurse?
- **Staying Healthy.** Does the health plan help people maintain good health and avoid illness? Does it give its doctors guidelines about how to provide appropriate preventive health services? Are members receiving tests and screenings as appropriate?

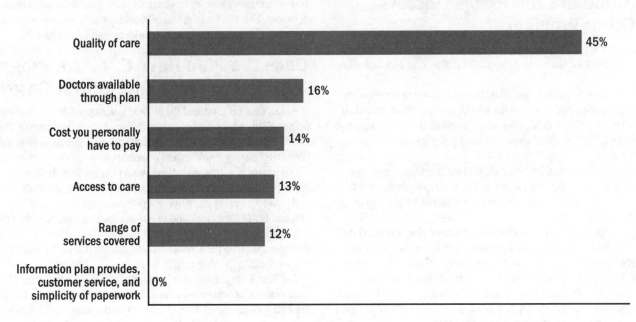

Which Features Members Consider Most Important

(Percentage of respondents who said feature was "most important")

Feature	Percentage
Quality of care	45%
Doctors available through plan	16%
Cost you personally have to pay	14%
Access to care	13%
Range of services covered	12%
Information plan provides, customer service, and simplicity of paperwork	0%

- **Getting Better.** How well does the health plan care for people when they become sick? How does the health plan evaluate new medical procedures, drugs, and devices to ensure that patients have access to safe and effective care?
- **Living with Illness.** How well does the health plan care for people with chronic conditions? Does the plan have programs in place to assist patients in managing chronic conditions like asthma? Do diabetics, who are at risk for blindness, receive eye exams as needed?

Based on its review, NCQA assigns one of the following accreditation levels, listed in order of desirability, to each plan—

- Excellent
- Commendable
- Accredited
- Provisional
- Denied

Plans that have the top three designations were all judged by NCQA to meet "NCQA's rigorous requirements for consumer protection and quality improvement." Plans with "Provisional" status were judged to meet only some of these standards. Current information on NCQA accreditation status can be found in NCQA's online report card at *www.ncqa.org.*

JCAHO's accreditation levels are—

- Accredited with commendation
- Accreditation with full standards compliance
- Accreditation with requirements for improvement
- Conditional accreditation
- Provisional accreditation
- Preliminary denial of accreditation
- Adverse decision, in appeal
- Accreditation denied

Current information on JCAHO accreditation status can be found in the "Quality Check" area of the JCAHO website at *www.jcaho.org.*

How Good are the Plan's Doctors and Other Providers?

Looking behind the overall ratings of plans to more specific aspects of performance, a key ingredient is the quality of a plan's doctors and other providers.

On our survey of physicians, we asked the doctors to rate the "quality of primary physicians affiliated with the HMO," the "quality of specialists affiliated with the HMO," and the "quality of hospitals doctors can refer to within the HMO." Results from these questions are given on the Plan Ratings table.

The survey of members asked for ratings of the member's "personal doctor or nurse" and asked for ratings of "the specialist you saw most often in the past 12 months." Results from these questions are also given on the Plan Ratings table.

In addition, the Plan Ratings table shows how each plan was rated by members on "how well doctors communicate." This is a composite of answers on four questions. It shows the percentage of times each plan's members, when asked about the last 12 months, reported that their doctors or other health providers "usually" or "always": listened carefully to them; explained things in a way they could understand; showed respect for what they had to say; and spent enough time with them. Such

communication is critical to good care. In many cases, the most important information to help diagnosis comes from the patient's own description. If a doctor doesn't listen well, this key information source may be lost. And it is also essential that the doctor explain well. Understanding what is wrong and what to expect enables you to monitor your care, avoid or recognize drug errors and other care mistakes, and help your doctor judge whether the current care strategy is working. Moreover, without a full understanding of what your care options are, you can't give informed consent to treatment.

If a plan's doctors and hospitals are rated high by the measures on the Plan Ratings table, your chances of finding good doctors are good even if you are not especially selective within the plan. On the other hand, even if a plan's doctors and hospitals generally get low ratings, you might be able to find good ones by choosing carefully.

On the other hand, you are not likely to have the benefit of the very best providers if the plan has few top providers on its list. Before enrolling in a plan, it's a good idea to check the provider list to see if doctors and hospitals you know to be outstanding are affiliated. Possible resources for identifying top-quality doctors and hospitals are our *Guide to Top Doctors* and *Consumers' Guide to Hospitals*. You can order online access to these resources or order them as printed books at *www.checkbook.org.* You will find that some plans have arranged for a much broader selection of top-quality providers than others have.

Does the Plan Have Effective Programs to Help Providers Give Better Care?

A plan that has recruited the highest quality providers is likely to deliver good care regardless of any other efforts it might make. But whatever the quality of its providers, a plan can still improve results with plan-sponsored quality improvement programs.

Our survey of physicians asked about plan features designed to help doctors provide the best possible care. The survey asked doctors to rate each "HMO's quality improvement programs and systems to help doctors practice better medicine" and to rate the "support services the HMO provides to help doctors follow up with patients." The results are on the Plan Ratings table. In general, plans rated relatively low on these measures, but some plans got high grades.

The Plan Ratings table also has another important indicator of each plan's quality improvement efforts. It reports whether each plan distinguished itself as one of the best (or one of the worst) on a number of direct measures of the actual care given to patients. We looked at 11 measures developed under the leadership of the National Committee for Quality Assurance. These measures are—

- Adolescent immunization status—the percentage of adolescent plan members who had received recommended hepatitis B, chicken pox, and other immunizations by their 13th birthday.
- Childhood immunization status—the percentage of child plan members who had received recommended diphtheria/pertussis/tetanus, polio, mumps/measles/rubella, and other immunizations by age two.
- Chlamydia screening—the percentage of sexually active women age 16 to 26 who had been screened for chlamydia, the most common sexually transmitted disease in the U.S.
- Breast cancer screening—the percentage of women age 52 to 69 who had had a mammogram to check for breast cancer within the past two years.
- Cervical cancer screening—the percentage of women age 21 to 64 who had had a Pap test to check for cervical cancer within the past three years.
- Beta blocker treatment after a heart attack—the percentage of plan members who were discharged from a hospital after surviving a heart attack who had received a prescription for beta blockers, a type of medication that has been shown to lower the risk of having another heart attack by lowering blood pressure and reducing how hard the heart has to work.
- Cholesterol management—the average of two percentages for plan members hospitalized for heart attack, bypass surgery, or angioplasty: (1) the percentage who had received screening for LDL-C ("bad" cholesterol) between 60 and 365 days after discharge; and (2) the percentage who had LDL-C levels controlled to less than 130 mg/dL during the same time period.
- Controlling high blood pressure—the percentage of members 46 to 85 years old who were previously diagnosed with high blood pressure who had had a blood pressure reading in the study period below certain danger thresholds, thus reducing the risk of heart disease, stroke, and kidney failure.
- Comprehensive diabetes care—for diabetic members, the average of six percentages relating to whether they had received appropriate tests and exams.
- Use of appropriate medications for people with asthma age five to 56—the percentage of people with asthma, the most common chronic childhood disease, who had been prescribed appropriate medications.
- Follow-up after hospitalization for mental illness—the percentage of members age six and older who had been hospitalized for selected mental disorders and who had been seen on an outpatient basis by a mental health provider within 30 days after discharge.

The Plan Ratings table indicates on which, if any, of these measures each plan scored at least as well as the best 25 percent of all plans for which we have data and on which, if any, measures its scores were among the worst 25 percent.

You might not have a strong interest in your plan's performance on most of the prevention and screening measures. The fact that a plan gets few of its women members to have Pap tests, for instance, doesn't say you personally would have a problem getting one. You might reasonably be more concerned with whether you can easily get the prevention and screening services if you want them. It is relevant to know that a plan can focus successful efforts on getting screening and prevention done. Success with such efforts might bode well for a plan's ability to conduct

other quality improvement programs on aspects of care that are not within your control. And some of the measures—like the beta blocker measure and the diabetes measure—tell you directly about aspects of care over which you have relatively little control.

But before putting too much weight on plans' performance on the 11 direct measures of care highlighted on the Plan Ratings table, you should keep in mind that these measures address only a tiny fraction of the activities of health care; unfortunately, developing and collecting data on measures of this kind is difficult and costly, so what is available now is limited. It is possible that a plan's performance on a short list of publicly reported measures may not reflect the overall quality of care within the plan; some plans may focus only on these publicly reported activities without addressing the full range of possible quality improvement opportunities.

Does the Plan Have Rules or Restrictions That Might Obstruct Good Care?

Just as plans can run programs to improve the quality of care, they might also have policies and practices that stand in the way of providers' abilities to deliver good care. These policies and practices—often motivated by a desire to cut costs—have brought HMOs intense criticism, and are one reason behind the pressure for legislation to protect health plan members.

Doctors have a first-hand look at obstructions some plans put in the way of care. The Plan Ratings table gives results on four questions we asked the doctors we surveyed with regard to such possible obstructions. We asked the doctors to rate plans on—

- Policies/practices affecting the ability of patients to see appropriate specialists;
- Policies/practices affecting the ability of patients to get appropriate and timely tests and treatments;
- Policies/practices affecting the ability of patients to get appropriate prescription drugs; and
- Incentives the HMO has created related to the quality of care doctors provide.

The Plan Ratings table shows the percentage of doctors who rated each plan "good," "very good," or "excellent." Even bearing in mind that some doctors may resent plans for financial reasons (plan restrictions on tests and treatments, for example, might reduce the doctors' income), the scores of many plans are surprisingly low.

On the Plan Ratings table, you will also find results for two important member survey measures of plan restrictions on care—the percent of members who said they had had "a big problem" getting referrals, tests, or treatment and the percentage who said they had not any problems getting referrals, tests, or treatment. For these two measures, we averaged the scores for three questions from the survey. Those three questions asked members whether in the last 12 months they had had "a big problem," "a small problem," or "not a problem"—

- Getting a referral to a specialist that you needed to see;
- Getting the care you or a doctor believed was necessary; and
- With delays in health care while you waited for approval from your health plan.

You will, of course, prefer plans where a high percentage of members have had no problem at all. But it is even more important to avoid plans where members have had a "big" problem. Presumably, any obstacle to

Challenges in Measuring Health Care Quality

The Plan Ratings table gives you valuable information to improve your odds of choosing a health plan that will give you high quality care and service. But you might reasonably ask for even stronger evidence telling you which plan is most likely to keep you alive and return you to good health if you have a serious medical problem. The information available on health plan quality is much better today than it was even ten years ago. But it is not all one would hope for.

Information on Results

For decades, there has been talk among those interested in measuring health plan quality about evaluating plans based on "outcomes." The idea is to judge HMOs by results—for example, how well a plan does in helping members be able to carry on a normal social life; perform basic activities of daily living (climbing stairs, bathing, etc.); and avoid missed days at work, pain, or death. Let's examine the possibilities of such outcome measurement.

One possible way to look at outcomes is to measure *changes* in members' health status or ability to function over a period of time. To focus on *plan-caused* differences more sharply, we might look specifically at outcomes for patients who have a particular disease—say, breast cancer—or who have been given a particular procedure—say, heart bypass surgery or hip replacement surgery. Are they alive, how do they feel, and how well can they function months and years after diagnosis or treatment?

Measuring plan-caused outcomes even in such cases is exceedingly difficult, however, for several reasons, including—

- The time required to observe results. For instance, if we must wait five years or 10 years to judge the success of a cancer treatment, the results might come in too late to be useful. By then, a plan might have completely changed its way of treating this type of cancer.
- The sample sizes required. Fortunately, many serious diseases don't hit large numbers of individuals each year. But that means reaching statistically reliable decisions about differences among plans may be difficult. If there are 200 new cervical cancer cases per year in each of two plans

with 250,000 members, a between-plan difference in survival rates might have to be greater than seven percentage points for us to be reasonably confident that the difference was not explained by luck alone. A seven percentage point difference might be rare.

- Problems in allowing for plan-to-plan differences in member characteristics and in the severity of cases. If plans differ in rates of long-term survival and in the ability of their patients to function following heart attacks, maybe the difference is explained by the lifestyle, the family support, or other characteristics of patients. Maybe there are differences in the severity of the heart attacks or in other health problems (say, diabetes or high blood pressure) the patients had. It might be possible to make adjustments for such differences when comparing plans, but for many types of cases, researchers don't yet understand what adjustments are appropriate.
- Lack of data. Suppose a key factor in predicting heart attack survival rates is whether the patient has had a previous heart attack. To compare survival rates for two plans, we would want to determine whether an equal proportion of each plan's patients had had previous heart attacks and, if not, to make appropriate adjustments. But plans might not know whether their patients had had previous heart attacks. This information might be contained in handwritten notes in each patient's medical record, located in the patient's physician's office. Collecting the information for all the cases in an entire plan might be very costly.

If doctors change to using computerized patient records, such data collection will be much easier. That's a very desirable change, but so far very few doctors are using computerized medical records and few plans are pushing doctors to start doing so. This is a major failing of the entire health care system—one that elected public officials and medical leaders should be moving aggressively to remedy.

There are other data problems also. For example, a low-quality doctor might not even record essential information. And terminology might differ from doctor to doctor and from plan to plan.

A key data problem is the lack of information on how patients are feeling and functioning after treatment. The way to get such information is to ask the patients. But most doctors and plans do not have procedures set up to get regular reports from patients days, months, and years after treatment. Even where patient followup surveys are done, response rates may be too low for the data to be useful, and pushing survey response rates up may be costly and may be annoying to patients.

In short, an ideal way to evaluate plan quality would be with measures of outcomes, but we won't have good outcome measures for many types of cases for years, and for others such measures will never be possible.

Can We Judge on Processes?

If we can't judge plans by results, or outcomes, can we judge by looking at what doctors *do*—do they give the right tests, prescribe the proper medication, counsel needed changes in patient behavior, etc.? For heart attack cases, for example, it is widely agreed that many patients should have beta blockers prescribed at the time of hospital discharge. We can compare plans by counting the percentage of heart attack patients for which this prescription was recorded.

But such "process" measures have their own problems, including the following—

- As a procedure becomes widely accepted, plan-to-plan variation may disappear. If we measure plans on whether doctors prescribe beta blockers for heart attack patients, it seems likely that nearly all doctors will soon get on board. That's good. But it means that the measure ceases to be an interesting basis for comparing plans. To the extent that we rely on process measures, we will need to be able to change the measures frequently.
- The large number of procedures. If we measure whether beta blockers are prescribed in heart attack cases, how about all the other procedures a doctor should—and shouldn't—do in these cases? Can we assume that doctors—and plans—that do one thing right do other things equally well?
- For many types of cases, we really don't

know what works. For decades, doctors prescribed Zantac and similar medications to relieve symptoms and foster healing of stomach ulcers. For a doctor to prescribe antibiotics would have been considered highly questionable. Now it is widely accepted that most stomach ulcers are caused by bacteria and should be treated with antibiotics. One can imagine just a few years ago an HMO performance evaluation system that would have measured plans based on whether doctors prescribed Zantac-like drugs. That would have rewarded physician behavior that did not contribute to the best outcomes—and might have slowed change to the more effective antibiotic treatment approach.

- The question of competence. If we decide, for example, that one of the processes we will measure is whether mammograms are given every two years to women over age 50, the measure may be meaningful, but we still won't know whether the mammograms are given and read competently or

followed up properly.

- Other problems. Even if we focus on measuring processes, we may still have sample size problems as we would with outcome measures; a small plan, for example, might not have many heart attack cases for which treatment with beta blockers is appropriate. We might also have problems allowing for differences in the characteristics of plan members; a plan that has less-educated members, for example, might have a bigger challenge than other plans in getting members to come in for mammograms. In addition, lack of data remains a serious concern. In the absence of computerized patient records, will it be necessary to read through hundreds of patient medical records in scores of doctors' offices to determine what percent of heart attack patients were given prescriptions for beta blockers or to determine whether certain of the patients not given beta blockers had medical conditions making beta blockers inappropriate?

The Prospects for Measurement

These complexities mean that comparing plans based on *either* results *or* medical care processes for some types of health problems will never be possible and that, for many types of health problems, implementing measures will take years and possibly be very costly.

Nonetheless, it is good that increasing policymaker interest and increasing resources are focused on measuring health plan quality—and that considerable progress has been made.

In coming years as you see various types of "report cards" that purport to report on quality, you'll want to keep in mind the inherent difficulties of quality measurement.

A key question that you will always need to ask is whether the data are independently audited. Data that are provided by plans without independent verification—or at least the possibility of verification with serious sanctions for misrepresentation—are useless.

getting care that a member believed might put his or her life or long-term well-being at risk would be reported as a "big" problem.

Often doctors are patients' main allies in fighting plans to authorize needed care. But sometimes doctors are the obstacle. In a basic HMO, your primary care doctor is your gatekeeper, who must authorize any care you will receive. As we have noted, some plans create financial incentives for doctors to keep care to a minimum. And regardless of such incentives, any single doctor might sometimes make bad decisions. You will not, therefore, want to be completely dependent on one doctor for your entire fate in the health care system.

It's important to be able to switch primary care doctors easily. That's no problem with indemnity plans or PPOs, but many HMOs require you to wait until the end of the month, and some allow you only one switch per year or limit you in other ways. Most of these restrictions are designed for the plan's administrative convenience rather than as a way to limit you. So the rules may be flexible. But you will want to check the restrictions on switching doctors in any plan you are considering. Ask a plan representative to show you the rules in its written materials. Surprisingly, some plans have different rules for different employer groups.

It is also important to be able to get a second opinion if you question a doctor's decision. Some plans *require* second opinions before they will authorize surgery or hospitalization and most plans are willing to pay for second opinions in such circumstances—where the second opinion might lead you to get less care and save the plan money. But you'll want also to be able to get a second opinion *paid for by the plan* if your primary care doctor has refused to authorize care. Ask plans to show you their written policies on this point. (Don't expect HMOs to pay for second opinions from nonplan doctors.)

How Convenient and Easy to Use Is the Plan's Care and Service?

In addition to the medical aspects of plan quality, you will also be interested in non-medical considerations. You will be able to judge some of these matters yourself. How convenient are the locations of the offices of the doctors you will have to use in a plan? How about the hospitals? How convenient are the doctors' or clinics' hours?

Other matters are better judged by the results of a member survey. On the Plan Ratings table, you will find plan-by-plan ratings on—

- Getting care quickly;
- Plan's customer service; and
- Plan's claims handling.

Each of these measures is a composite of responses to several questions. For example, the "getting care quickly" measure shows, with reference to the last 12 months, the percent of favorable answers on an "always," "usually," "sometimes," or "never" scale on four questions—

- "When you called during regular office hours, how often did you get the help or advice you needed?"
- "How often did you get an appointment for regular or routine health care as soon as you wanted?"
- "When you needed care right away for an illness or injury, how often did you get care as soon as you wanted?"
- "How often did you wait in the doctor's office or clinic more than 15 minutes past your appointment time to see the person you went to see?"

Plan Ratings

✓ means plan receives our top rating
Highest scores are in Blue
Lowest scores are in **Bold Italic**
"—" means no data

Footnotes are on page 56

	Doctors' overall rating of plan for patient care (% favorable)	Members' overall rating of plan (% favorable)	Key performance measures — Direct measures of actual care for which plan was among the best or worst plans (see codes below)* Best	Worst or not reported	Accreditation status**	"Big" problem getting referrals/tests/care	Called/wrote plan with complaint or problem
Average for all plans	57	60				9	20
Arizona							
Aetna U.S. Healthcare (Southern and western Arizona)	57	55	be	cf	Commendable	*12*	18
BlueCross BlueShield of Arizona (All or most of Arizona)	84	—	—	—	None	—	—
CIGNA HealthCare of Arizona (Parts of Arizona)	60	57	bcdefgij	None	Excellent	*13*	18
Health Net of Arizona (HMO) (Most of Arizona)	51	*49*	None	bcfghij	Commendable	—	—
Humana Health Plans (HMO) (Southern and western Arizona)	47	*50*	c	abdhij	None	*19*	23
Mayo Health Plan Arizona (Phoenix area)	96	—	—	—	None	—	—
PacifiCare of Arizona (HMO) (Phoenix and Tuscon areas)	*29*	*51*	k	ghj	Excellent	17	21
UnitedHealthcare of Arizona (All or most of Arizona)	75	—	—	—	JCAHO	—	—
Arkansas							
Aetna U.S. Healthcare (Crittenden County)	—	59	None	abcdefghijk	Accredited	—	—
✓ HealthLink (HMO) (Little Rock area and parts of Northern Arkansas)	71	66	—	—	None	4	13
HealthLink (POS) (Little Rock area and parts of Northern Arkansas)	71	65	—	—	None	6	20
UnitedHealthcare of Arkansas (Most of Arkansas)	—	60	None	aefghik	None	6	23
California							
Aetna U.S. Healthcare (Northern California)	55	*50*	af	cgk	Commendable	*14*	19
Aetna U.S. Healthcare (Most of Southern California)	54	56	afgh	cd	Commendable	*18*	17
Aetna U.S. Healthcare (San Diego County)	61	61	abdehi	None	Excellent	*13*	13
Blue Cross of California/California Care (Most or all of California)	*45*	*51*	None	cjk	Commendable	15	12
Blue Shield of California (Most of California)	54	*51*	None	bcdghijk	Commendable	—	—
CIGNA HealthCare of California (Most of California)	51	*51*	h	ck	Commendable	*19*	*27*
Health Net of California (Most of California)	48	57	a	cefgk	Commendable	*14*	17
HP of the Redwoods (HMO) (Lake, Marin, Mendocino, Sonoma cos)	*29*	59	ak	cg	Excellent	15	20
InterValley HP (LA, Orange, Riverside, San Bernardino, Ventura cos)	*44*	—	—	—	None	—	—
✓ Kaiser Permanente California (HMO) (Northern California)	95	58	bcfgik	h	Excellent	*13*	8
✓ Kaiser Permanente California (HMO) (Southern California)	84	62	abcgi	j	Commendable	*13*	11
Lifeguard (HMO) (Northern California)	62	60	de	None	Commendable	*13*	18
One Health Plan of CA (Bay Area, Fresno, Sacramento, and So. CA)	48	—	—	—	None	—	—
PacifiCare of California (Most of California)	*45*	*54*	ah	c	Commendable	16	17
Sharp Health Plan (HMO) (San Diego area)	68	55	—	—	None	15	17
UHP Healthcare (Los Angeles area)	*26*	—	—	—	JCAHO	—	—
Universal Care (HMO) (Southern California)	*41*	57	None	abcdefghijk	Commendable	16	18
Western Health Advantage (HMO) (Sacramento area)	69	68	—	—	None	10	15

*Assuring proper prevention and screening: a=Adolescent immunizations; b=Childhood immunizations; c=Chlamydia screening in sexually active women; d=Breast cancer screening; e=Cervical cancer screening. **Assuring proper treatment:** f=Beta blocker treatment after a heart attack; g=Cholesterol management (two measures); h=Controlling high blood pressure; i=Comprehensive diabetes care (six measures); j=Use of appropriate asthma medication; k=Followup after hospitalization for mental illness. "Best" or "worst" indicates plan's scores were in either the top or bottom 25 percent of benchmark plans.

Detailed performance measures

Ability of patients to see appropriate specialists	Ability of patients to get needed tests and treatments	Ability of patients to get appropriate drugs	Plan's programs to help doctors give better care	How plan helps doctors follow up with patients	Incentives plan gives doctors affecting quality of care	Quality of primary care physicians affiliated with plan	Quality of specialists affiliated with plan	Quality of hospitals doctors can refer to within the plan	Number of doctors rating plan on the survey	Overall health care	Personal doctors	Specialist doctors	No problem getting referrals/tests/care	Getting care quickly	How well doctors communicate	Plan's customer service	Plan's claims processing	Estimated cost index for single person	Plan's phone number
56	56	52	42	36	30	72	76	78		73	75	77	79	78	90	67	81	$1.00	800-999-9999
56	55	47	46	37	24	77	75	81	127	67	72	73	73	73	87	65	79	$0.88	800-323-9930
81	82	78	63	57	37	88	93	91	134	–	–	–	–	–	–	–	–	–	877-864-4899
52	58	51	50	52	36	71	74	81	116	63	68	69	73	74	84	64	81	–	800-832-3211
47	51	37	38	40	27	68	67	71	90	60	70	72	–	67	87	69	85	$0.99	800-909-3447
46	47	40	39	34	21	61	60	68	104	60	67	67	65	69	87	60	78	–	800-448-6262
94	94	91	80	75	62	96	96	95	95	–	–	–	–	–	–	–	–	–	800-335-6296
35	41	21	27	26	10	54	51	59	102	65	73	70	65	69	86	63	80	$0.92	800-347-8600
75	70	63	56	53	38	81	85	85	131	–	–	–	–	–	–	–	–	–	602-664-2676
–	–	–	–	–	–	–	–	–	–	68	79	75	–	67	86	69	81	$0.90	800-323-9930
69	74	73	38	35	26	81	83	86	63	80	76	85	84	80	91	67	89	–	800-624-2356
69	74	73	38	35	26	81	83	86	63	76	76	81	81	84	91	63	85	–	800-624-2356
–	–	–	–	–	–	–	–	–	–	77	78	75	84	81	93	61	76	–	501-664-7700
57	60	57	41	33	31	80	81	83	152	68	70	72	72	75	88	62	73	–	800-323-9930
60	57	51	43	40	29	70	74	73	243	65	71	68	66	68	85	61	71	$0.83	800-323-9930
61	61	44	38	37	26	77	79	86	86	69	74	70	72	75	89	65	82	–	800-323-9930
51	50	44	36	31	24	68	72	73	389	60	64	72	69	71	85	64	82	$0.87	800-333-0912
56	54	50	42	37	30	72	78	76	490	64	68	70	–	70	84	61	78	$0.92	800-200-3242
56	55	45	38	34	27	70	75	75	434	54	66	68	62	67	82	62	71	$0.96	800-832-3211
53	51	43	38	34	26	69	75	73	535	67	71	72	70	72	87	64	80	$0.94	800-909-3447
37	44	42	27	23	13	70	64	59	28	76	78	82	69	81	91	67	89	–	800-248-2070
45	47	34	35	30	20	58	61	59	93	–	–	–	–	–	–	–	–	–	800-251-8191
93	93	96	95	94	91	97	96	95	373	64	70	72	76	76	84	76	–	$0.89	800-464-4000
85	84	82	84	82	80	87	88	87	235	65	74	71	75	72	84	78	–	$0.93	800-464-4000
64	64	58	50	40	34	79	81	85	150	68	69	76	73	76	89	64	82	–	800-995-0380
56	55	47	36	31	28	67	74	71	180	–	–	–	–	–	–	–	–	–	800-663-8081
48	48	33	33	28	24	65	71	70	489	64	70	70	66	71	85	65	79	$0.76	800-624-8822
63	64	51	50	46	35	78	83	79	59	67	73	73	70	72	88	67	78	–	800-359-2002
44	38	26	24	19	25	43	49	46	89	–	–	–	–	–	–	–	–	–	800-847-1222
49	49	35	29	30	27	56	65	62	160	64	72	71	66	69	84	65	71	$0.71	800-635-6668
68	64	60	46	50	44	75	89	88	39	71	73	75	73	72	88	67	87	$0.89	888-227-5942

Accreditation status with NCQA (1/2002) is shown. Accreditation status with JCAHO (1/2002) is shown as follows: JCAHO=With commendation or with full standards compliance; JCAHO=With requirements for improvement. **Accreditation with the American

Accreditation HealthCare Commission is shown as: AAHC. None=No accreditation action reported by any of the three accrediting organizations.

Plan Ratings

✓ means plan receives our top rating
Highest scores are in Blue
Lowest scores are in *Bold Italic*
"–" means no data

Footnotes are on page 56

	Doctors' overall rating of plan for patient care (% favorable)	Members' overall rating of plan (% favorable)	Direct measures of actual care for which plan was among the best or worst plans (see codes below)*		Accreditation status**	% of members who had a problem (lower is better)	
Key performance measures			Best	Worst or not reported		"Big" problem getting referrals/tests/care	Called/wrote plan with complaint or problem
Average for all plans	57	60				9	20
Colorado							
Aetna U.S. Healthcare (Front Range area)	57	*53*	ef	ck	None	10	*16*
CIGNA HealthCare of Colorado (Front Range area)	61	56	acdfhk	None	Commendable	*11*	23
Community Health Plan of the Rockies (Front Range area)	*29*	–	–		None	–	–
Denver Health Medical Plan (HMO) (Denver)	–	62	ak	bcdeghij	Commendable	–	–
HMO Colorado (Most or all of Colorado)	55	*47*	f	bceghij	Commendable	*13*	21
✓ Kaiser Permanente Colorado (Denver and Colorado Springs areas)	80	60	abcdeghijk	None	Excellent	10	10
One Health Plan of Colorado (Front Range area)	74	–	–	–	None	–	–
PacifiCare of Colorado (Front Range area)	*26*	*52*	aek	h	Commendable	*12*	19
✓ Rocky Mountain HMO (Most of Colorado)	60	61	adefj	None	Excellent	7	20
UnitedHealthcare of Colorado (HMO) (Front Range area)	75	60	–	–	Commendable	–	–
Connecticut							
Aetna U.S. Healthcare (All or most of Connecticut)	*43*	*48*	bhjk	None	Excellent	9	21
✓ Anthem Blue Cross and Blue Shield (All or most of Connecticut)	78	65	bcefhjk	None	Excellent	5	17
CIGNA HealthCare of Connecticut (All of Connecticut)	53	57	bdj	None	Commendable	5	*24*
✓ ConnectiCare (All or most of Connecticut)	60	68	bcdefjk	h	Excellent	7	16
First Choice Health Plan (All or most of Connecticut)	51	–	–	–	None	–	–
Health Net of the Northeast[1] (All or most of Connecticut)	*44*	71	–	–	None	4	17
✓ Health New England (Northern Connecticut)	–	73	acfk	hi	Excellent	5	12
HMO New England (All or most of Connecticut)	50	–	–	–	None	–	–
MedSpan Health Options (All or most of Connecticut)	63	–	–	–	None	–	–
Oxford Health Plans (All or most of Connecticut)	*46*	59	degj	hi	Commendable	*11*	19
UnitedHealthcare of New York (Fairfield County)	66	*54*	c	dehik	Commendable	8	*28*
Delaware							
✓ Aetna U.S. Healthcare (Northern Delaware)	56	68	bi	None	Excellent	5	14
AmeriHealth HMO of Delaware (All of Delaware)	51	59	a	cehj	Excellent	8	*24*
BlueCross BlueShield of Delaware (All of Delaware)	–	68	ak	bcghij	Excellent	–	–
CIGNA HealthCare of Delaware (All of Delaware)	*42*	*47*	abch	None	Excellent	*13*	27
Coventry Health Care (All of Delaware)	*36*	63	acd	gjk	None	6	*28*
Delmarva Health Plan (All of Delaware)	–	70	None	ghj	None	5	17
Keystone Health Plan East (All or most of Delaware)	*40*	65	abi	cde	Excellent	8	13
Optimum Choice (All of Delaware)	54	62	b	f	Excellent	9	16

*Assuring proper prevention and screening: a=Adolescent immunizations; b=Childhood immunizations; c=Chlamydia screening in sexually active women; d=Breast cancer screening; e=Cervical cancer screening. Assuring proper treatment: f=Beta blocker treatment after a heart attack; g=Cholesterol management (two measures); h=Controlling high blood pressure; i=Comprehensive diabetes care (six measures); j=Use of appropriate asthma medication; k=Followup after hospitalization for mental illness. "Best" or "worst" indicates plan's scores were in either the top or bottom 25 percent of benchmark plans.

Detailed performance measures

Ratings by doctors (% favorable)										Ratings by members (% favorable)									
Ability of patients to see appropriate specialists	Ability of patients to get needed tests and treatments	Ability of patients to get appropriate drugs	Plan's programs to help doctors give better care	How plan helps doctors follow up with patients	Incentives plan gives doctors affecting quality of care	Quality of primary care physicians affiliated with plan	Quality of specialists affiliated with plan	Quality of hospitals doctors can refer to within the plan	Number of doctors rating plan on the survey	Overall health care	Personal doctors	Specialist doctors	No problem getting referrals/tests/care	Getting care quickly	How well doctors communicate	Plan's customer service	Plan's claims processing	Estimated cost index for single person	Plan's phone number
56	56	52	42	36	30	72	76	78		73	75	77	79	78	90	67	81	$1.00	800-999-9999
60	57	58	39	39	37	82	85	86	81	71	74	76	78	82	91	64	81	–	800-323-9930
63	58	47	42	36	29	81	85	89	82	69	70	77	73	77	88	61	82	–	800-832-3211
34	28	42	26	20	21	48	58	66	52	–	–	–	–	–	–	–	–		800-995-3220
–	–	–	–	–	–	–	–	–	–	77	82	73	–	73	93	66	75	–	303-436-6000
59	61	59	45	36	38	74	81	80	78	67	66	74	72	78	90	58	78	–	800-334-6557
69	75	82	74	83	70	83	81	81	51	66	74	67	82	78	88	73	–	$0.92	888-681-7878
77	66	68	47	33	33	77	82	83	62	–	–	–	–	–	–	–	–	–	800-663-8081
34	33	28	26	20	20	65	61	64	86	71	72	77	73	80	89	60	85	$1.00	800-877-9777
63	58	64	44	33	38	77	75	80	70	75	75	76	84	83	92	63	87	$1.29	800-843-0719
82	76	77	57	54	48	92	81	93	85	70	–	–	–	–	–	–	–	–	303-267-3300
47	47	41	27	25	15	78	78	84	185	72	73	74	78	81	90	62	73	–	800-323-9930
80	78	64	47	41	29	92	91	91	188	81	79	83	89	83	93	72	87	–	800-545-0948
54	55	42	35	28	23	81	80	84	166	78	75	80	80	83	93	62	79	–	800-832-3211
64	59	50	45	36	24	82	81	82	170	79	77	80	86	84	93	75	90	$0.94	800-251-7722
63	54	49	27	16	18	70	75	86	35	–	–	–	–	–	–	–	–	–	800-288-5441
49	41	36	27	25	13	77	76	83	177	80	78	81	87	83	91	70	87	$1.20	800-909-3447
–	–	–	–	–	–	–	–	–	–	78	78	79	90	85	92	80	92	$1.11	800-842-4464
51	61	52	40	26	21	80	81	79	30	–	–	–	–	–	–	–	–	–	800-331-0150
69	70	57	40	30	25	84	82	82	125	–	–	–	–	–	–	–	–	–	800-767-4008
47	50	38	32	27	17	71	74	75	158	77	79	79	77	81	91	63	80	–	800-444-6222
69	68	60	48	40	37	79	78	79	419	67	73	72	82	75	90	65	71	–	800-339-5380
58	55	41	39	33	25	80	89	86	124	77	82	82	87	82	93	72	86	$1.17	800-323-9930
48	49	41	34	30	22	76	79	78	155	73	73	72	82	82	91	65	78	–	302-777-6400
–	–	–	–	–	–	–	–	–	–	73	72	79	–	82	90	73	85	–	800-572-4400
42	40	35	35	27	29	68	71	79	41	69	67	78	75	78	89	59	71	–	800-832-3211
42	37	40	30	14	18	66	69	70	47	75	72	78	87	82	90	65	77	–	800-833-7423
–	–	–	–	–	–	–	–	–	–	78	79	83	90	81	93	76	89	–	800-334-3427
41	37	32	28	23	18	73	76	77	296	73	78	75	83	80	91	73	87	$1.01	800-555-1514
54	51	52	37	32	26	72	76	76	314	69	68	77	79	75	88	70	83	–	800-331-2102

Accreditation status with NCQA (1/2002) is shown. Accreditation status with JCAHO (1/2002) is shown as follows: JCAHO=With commendation or with full standards compliance; JCAHO=With requirements for improvement. **Accreditation with the American

Accreditation HealthCare Commission is shown as: AAHC. None=No accreditation action reported by any of the three accrediting organizations.

Plan Ratings

✓ means plan receives our top rating
Highest scores are in Blue
Lowest scores are in *Bold Italic*
"—" means no data

Footnotes are on page 56

	Doctors' overall rating of plan for patient care (% favorable)	Members' overall rating of plan (% favorable)	Direct measures of actual care for which plan was among the best or worst plans (see codes below)*		Accreditation status**	% of members who had a problem (lower is better)	
			Best	Worst or not reported		"Big" problem getting referrals/tests/care	Called/wrote plan with complaint or problem
Average for all plans	57	60				9	20
District of Columbia							
Aetna U.S. Healthcare (District of Columbia)	*39*	*48*	bfh	cg	Commendable	*12*	23
Capital Care/CareFirst (District of Columbia)	63	58	bdj	h	Excellent	9	23
CIGNA HealthCare Mid-Atlantic (District of Columbia)	50	*48*	bch	i	Excellent	*13*	22
Kaiser Foundation Health Plan Mid-Atlantic States (HMO) (DC)	56	60	abcef	None	Commendable	10	*13*
M.D. IPA (District of Columbia)	50	70	bhj	f	Excellent	7	20
Optimum Choice (District of Columbia)	54	62	b	f	Excellent	9	16
Preferred Health Network[2] (District of Columbia)	70	*51*	—	—	None	6	29
UnitedHealthcare of the Mid-Atlantic (HMO) (District of Columbia)	57	*54*	—	—	JCAHO	5	25
Florida							
Aetna U.S. Healthcare (Most of Florida)	60	60	agh	dk	Commendable	*11*	19
AvMed (HMO) (Most of Florida)	*46*	63	None	bghk	Commendable[3]	*12*	23
Beacon Health Plans[4] (South Florida)	*34*	*50*	—	—	None	*18*	—
✓ Capital Health Plan (HMO) (Tallahassee area)	—	76	abcdegik	None	Excellent	6	9
CIGNA HealthCare of Florida[4] (Most of Florida)	65	58	abcegh	None	Commendable	9	—
Florida 1st Health Plans[4] (Central Florida)	65	63	—	—	None	6	—
✓ Florida Health Care Plans[4] (Flagler and Volusia counties)	72	69	—	—	JCAHO	9	—
Foundation Health (South, central, and western Florida)	*39*	*45*	None	bcghijk	Commendable	—	—
Health First Health Plans (HMO) (Brevard and Indian River counties)	68	61	abj	ci	Commendable	10	17
Health Options (Central, eastern, and southern Florida)	58	56	acgi	k	Excellent	*11*	16
Health Options (Northern and western Florida)	57	56	abeghi	k	Commendable	10	18
Healthplan Southeast[4] (Gainesville, Ocala, Pensacola, Tallahasse)	—	*53*	—	—	Commendable	10	—
Humana Health Plans (HMO) (Central Florida)	52	*49*	ag	cdej	Commendable[3]	*15*	25
Humana Health Plans (HMO) (Northern Florida)	—	*48*	d	cej	Commendable[3]	*15*	29
Humana Health Plans (HMO) (South Florida)	*37*	56	ah	bcejk	Commendable[3]	*15*	19
Humana Health Plans (HMO) (Tampa Bay area)	*43*	*51*	ab	cejk	Commendable[3]	*16*	26
JMH Health Plan[4] (Broward and Miami-Dade counties)	59	66	—	—	None	*12*	—
Neighborhood Health Partnership (South Florida)	47	55	None	aefghijk	Commendable	*15*	19
One Health Plan[4] (Fort Myers, Orlando, South Florida, Tampa Bay)	69	*52*	—	—	None	14	—
Preferred Medical Plan[4] (Broward and Miami-Dade counties)	49	62	—	—	None	9	—
Total Health Choice[4] (South, central, and eastern Florida)	*39*	60	—	—	None	*16*	—
✓ UnitedHealthcare of Florida[4] (Most of Florida)	74	74	—	—	JCAHO	4	—
WellCare HMO[4] (South, central, and western Florida)	*36*	*48*	—	—	None	*16*	—

*Assuring proper prevention and screening: a=Adolescent immunizations; b=Childhood immunizations; c=Chlamydia screening in sexually active women; d=Breast cancer screening; e=Cervical cancer screening. Assuring proper treatment: f=Beta blocker treatment after a heart attack; g=Cholesterol management (two measures); h=Controlling high blood pressure; i=Comprehensive diabetes care (six measures); j=Use of appropriate asthma medication; k=Followup after hospitalization for mental illness. "Best" or "worst" indicates plan's scores were in either the top or bottom 25 percent of benchmark plans.

Detailed performance measures

Ratings by doctors (% favorable)										Ratings by members (% favorable)									
Ability of patients to see appropriate specialists	Ability of patients to get needed tests and treatments	Ability of patients to get appropriate drugs	Plan's programs to help doctors give better care	How plan helps doctors follow up with patients	Incentives plan gives doctors affecting quality of care	Quality of primary care physicians affiliated with plan	Quality of specialists affiliated with plan	Quality of hospitals doctors can refer to within the plan	Number of doctors rating plan on the survey	Overall health care	Personal doctors	Specialist doctors	No problem getting referrals/tests/care	Getting care quickly	How well doctors communicate	Plan's customer service	Plan's claims processing	Estimated cost index for single person	Plan's phone number
56	56	52	42	36	30	72	76	78		73	75	77	79	78	90	67	81	$1.00	800-999-9999
39	38	41	29	20	18	62	66	75	351	68	71	74	76	76	89	60	74	$1.08	800-323-9930
62	62	59	44	37	33	78	81	82	305	71	72	77	80	77	87	65	80	$1.02	800-296-5555
50	50	45	31	28	21	65	68	72	254	64	68	72	74	76	88	65	76	–	800-832-3211
53	52	64	55	48	46	60	64	77	179	63	73	64	78	77	85	74	64	$0.86	800-777-7902
50	49	51	34	31	25	69	73	73	319	73	71	75	84	78	90	75	87	$0.96	800-782-1966
54	51	52	37	32	26	72	76	76	314	69	68	77	79	75	88	70	83	–	800-331-2102
69	66	58	38	32	32	74	79	80	135	72	77	78	81	75	91	55	69	–	800-422-1996
63	60	49	35	29	25	67	73	78	223	73	78	77	84	77	89	57	71	–	800-368-1680
60	59	54	40	34	30	73	76	78	440	70	78	75	77	74	88	67	85	–	800-323-9930
44	43	40	30	28	25	57	59	66	298	68	65	70	71	71	86	74	82	$1.00	800-882-8633
38	33	33	25	22	17	45	49	57	211	73	78	81	62	66	90	61	–	–	800-850-0979
–	–	–	–	–	–	–	–	–	–	78	80	80	86	80	92	80	94	$0.96	850-383-3311
64	63	54	46	44	37	74	77	80	417	66	70	74	76	70	83	67	–	–	800-832-3211
62	66	54	43	41	37	75	78	82	88	73	78	77	80	75	87	67	–	–	800-226-3155
71	63	63	60	49	34	78	78	76	43	74	78	78	80	77	86	73	–	–	800-232-0578
42	42	38	28	25	21	49	53	60	285	57	61	64	–	65	80	60	72	$0.71	800-441-5501
57	55	57	41	28	21	63	75	81	31	68	68	70	80	73	88	76	89	–	800-716-7737
56	55	51	43	35	26	61	67	72	280	65	69	69	74	67	84	67	85	–	800-964-6371
52	54	48	43	33	29	74	74	78	135	66	70	72	76	75	88	62	80	–	800-964-6371
–	–	–	–	–	–	–	–	–	–	79	81	85	71	77	90	54	–	–	800-833-2169
51	43	42	35	34	26	52	64	68	54	58	63	69	67	68	80	64	76	–	800-448-6262
–	–	–	–	–	–	–	–	–	–	63	74	73	69	73	86	60	73	–	800-448-6262
39	37	40	31	29	22	48	55	63	260	59	66	72	70	66	81	69	72	–	800-448-6262
42	42	28	36	27	32	53	66	69	74	61	67	76	71	69	85	65	79	–	800-448-6262
57	50	52	35	40	36	63	70	73	97	77	86	83	71	63	89	73	–	–	305-575-3700
49	44	40	30	27	25	54	57	63	199	68	77	81	69	66	86	67	71	–	800-354-0222
67	65	60	47	40	49	72	72	75	64	64	70	79	69	67	86	57	–	–	800-663-8081
44	40	44	34	33	28	49	52	59	73	72	86	76	75	63	85	72	–	–	800-767-5551
42	40	35	24	26	24	39	43	53	84	71	84	81	68	66	84	68	–	–	305-408-5823
76	74	68	57	50	44	79	83	85	471	80	85	81	87	75	92	70	–	–	954-858-4000
40	35	33	26	22	22	43	46	58	222	68	74	73	68	68	85	60	–	–	800-960-2530

Accreditation status with NCQA (1/2002) is shown. Accreditation status with JCAHO (1/2002) is shown as follows: JCAHO=With commendation or with full standards compliance; JCAHO=With requirements for improvement. **Accreditation with the American Accreditation HealthCare Commission is shown as: AAHC. None=No accreditation action reported by any of the three accrediting organizations.**

Plan Ratings

✓ means plan receives our top rating
Highest scores are in Blue
Lowest scores are in *Bold Italic*
"—" means no data

Footnotes are on page 56

	Doctors' overall rating of plan for patient care (% favorable)	Members' overall rating of plan (% favorable)	Direct measures of actual care for which plan was among the best or worst plans (see codes below)* — Best	Direct measures ... — Worst or not reported	Accreditation status**	"Big" problem getting referrals/tests/care	Called/wrote plan with complaint or problem
Average for all plans	57	60				9	20
Georgia							
Aetna U.S. Healthcare (Athens, Atlanta, and Augusta areas)	*43*	*54*	be	i	Excellent	*11*	21
BlueCross BlueShield of Georgia[2] (Most of Georgia)	54	62	bh	k	Excellent	9	18
CIGNA HealthCare of Georgia (Northern Georgia)	52	–	bc	dfi	Commendable	–	–
Coventry Health Care of Georgia (Atlanta area)	49	–	–	–	None	–	–
Humana Health Plans (HMO) (Atlanta area)	52	*45*	None	cdi	None	*17*	*30*
✓ Kaiser Permanente Georgia (HMO) (Atlanta area)	63	66	bcdegik	j	Excellent	9	13
One Health Plan of Georgia (Atlanta and Macon areas)	57	–	–	–	None	–	–
UnitedHealthcare of Georgia (Most of Georgia)	69	59	None	abcfghij	Commendable	–	–
Guam							
PacifiCare Asia Pacific (HMO) (Guam)	–	67	–		None	7	13
Hawaii							
✓ Health Plan Hawaii (HMO) (Most of Hawaii)	–	71	ach	df	Excellent	8	9
✓ HMSA (All of Hawaii)	–	78	–	–	Excellent	2	8
✓ Kaiser Permanente Hawaii (HMO) (Most of Hawaii)	–	72	abcdfgij	h	Excellent	10	8
Idaho							
✓ Group Health Cooperative (HMO) (Northern Idaho)	71	60	aceijk	b	Excellent	10	9
Group Health Options (Northern Idaho)	–	57	aceijk	None	None	10	17
Group Health Options (POS) (Northern Idaho)	–	*53*	cgk	bh	None	10	18
Intermountain Health Care (Southern Idaho)	93	61	–	–	Commendable	–	–
Illinois							
Aetna U.S. Healthcare (Chicago area)	*43*	*46*	None	bcdeghik	Commendable	*11*	*29*
Aetna U.S. Healthcare (St. Louis area)	52	–	–	–	None	–	–
BlueCHOICE (St. Louis area)	*44*	57	None	cfgijk	Commendable	7	*16*
BlueChoice (POS) (Chicago, Rockford, Springfield, St. Louis areas)	–	55	None	bcefghj	Commendable	10	*29*
CIGNA HealthCare of Illinois (Most of Illinois)	58	55	ah	d	Commendable	*12*	23
✓ CIGNA HealthCare of St. Louis (St. Louis area)	74	63	abfh	None	Commendable	8	18
Group Health Plan (St. Louis area)	*38*	65	abj	ceik	None	9	*16*
✓ Health Alliance (Central and southern Illinois)	–	67	dhj	f	Excellent	8	*16*
✓ HealthLink (HMO) (Central and southern Illinois)	71	66			None	4	13
HealthLink (POS) (Central and southern Illinois)	71	65	–	–	None	6	20
HMO IL/BlueAdvantage (HMO) (Chi., Peor., Rockford, Sprgf'd, St. L)	58	56	a	bchj	Excellent	*11*	23
Humana Health Plan–Illinois (HMO) (Chicago area)	*45*	*54*	a	bcegik	Commendable	*11*	23

*Assuring proper prevention and screening: a=Adolescent immunizations; b=Childhood immunizations; c=Chlamydia screening in sexually active women; d=Breast cancer screening; e=Cervical cancer screening. Assuring proper treatment: f=Beta blocker treatment after a heart attack; g=Cholesterol management (two measures); h=Controlling high blood pressure; i=Comprehensive diabetes care (six measures); j=Use of appropriate asthma medication; k=Followup after hospitalization for mental illness. "Best" or "worst" indicates plan's scores were in either the top or bottom 25 percent of benchmark plans.

Detailed performance measures

Ratings by doctors (% favorable)										Ratings by members (% favorable)									
Ability of patients to see appropriate specialists	Ability of patients to get needed tests and treatments	Ability of patients to get appropriate drugs	Plan's programs to help doctors give better care	How plan helps doctors follow up with patients	Incentives plan gives doctors affecting quality of care	Quality of primary care physicians affiliated with plan	Quality of specialists affiliated with plan	Quality of hospitals doctors can refer to within the plan	Number of doctors rating plan on the survey	Overall health care	Personal doctors	Specialist doctors	No problem getting referrals/tests/care	Getting care quickly	How well doctors communicate	Plan's customer service	Plan's claims processing	Estimated cost index for single person	Plan's phone number
56	56	52	42	36	30	72	76	78		73	75	77	79	78	90	67	81	$1.00	800-999-9999
42	42	43	36	32	18	62	74	76	136	73	74	76	75	74	89	64	74	$0.94	800-323-9930
52	49	48	47	42	28	75	78	82	138	71	74	75	80	78	90	69	84	—	800-441-2273
49	45	39	41	35	22	71	77	78	125	—	—	—	—	—	—	—	—	—	800-832-3211
44	49	45	32	32	26	65	68	73	77	—	—	—	—	—	—	—	—	—	800-395-2545
54	55	48	31	23	20	66	69	70	71	57	61	77	67	72	82	57	63	—	800-448-6262
50	52	47	54	52	40	56	58	70	73	69	76	69	82	77	88	77	76	$0.85	800-611-1811
62	56	51	33	32	24	65	72	75	65	—	—	—	—	—	—	—	—	—	800-663-8081
70	69	57	59	39	35	72	77	77	121	76	77	76	—	76	89	65	75	—	404-982-8800
—	—	—	—	—	—	—	—	—	—	74	76	73	73	72	88	68	70	$1.04	671-647-3526
—	—	—	—	—	—	—	—	—	—	79	81	74	84	83	93	76	93	—	800-618-4672
—	—	—	—	—	—	—	—	—	—	87	87	84	91	89	96	77	95	$0.88	800-618-4672
—	—	—	—	—	—	—	—	—	—	75	77	75	82	80	92	76	—	$0.98	800-966-5955
66	63	67	78	60	47	79	79	78	59	69	72	73	80	81	90	72	84	$1.04[5]	888-901-4636
—	—	—	—	—	—	—	—	—	—	71	70	75	80	81	90	67	75	—	800-542-6312
—	—	—	—	—	—	—	—	—	—	68	71	73	78	79	92	66	77	—	800-542-6312
75	81	82	74	60	51	92	95	94	58	68	77	—	—	75	89	62	—	—	800-538-5038
43	40	42	31	30	26	70	76	70	192	64	72	69	76	76	89	65	63	—	800-323-9930
56	62	65	29	31	24	79	83	81	56	—	—	—	—	—	—	—	—	—	800-323-9930
52	52	57	33	24	28	74	85	80	52	74	76	76	84	81	92	64	86	$0.98	800-932-4480
—	—	—	—	—	—	—	—	—	—	73	75	75	76	78	90	60	75	—	800-654-7385
55	52	48	41	37	33	76	78	77	158	66	68	66	75	77	88	65	80	—	800-832-3211
70	71	60	40	35	21	85	91	91	57	75	71	78	81	82	91	69	89	—	800-832-3211
41	39	36	32	22	17	65	82	81	68	81	75	81	81	81	91	69	87	$1.18	800-755-3901
—	—	—	—	—	—	—	—	—	—	77	79	78	83	85	92	70	87	$1.13	800-851-3379
69	74	73	38	35	26	81	83	86	63	80	76	85	84	80	91	67	89	—	800-624-2356
69	74	73	38	35	26	81	83	86	63	76	76	81	81	84	91	63	85	—	800-624-2356
54	54	55	46	39	35	74	76	76	189	68	71	66	76	76	88	62	70	—	800-892-2803
40	43	37	31	28	30	66	73	74	154	66	71	73	78	75	87	65	65	—	800-448-6262

Accreditation status with NCQA (1/2002) is shown. Accreditation status with JCAHO (1/2002) is shown as follows: JCAHO=With commendation or with full standards compliance; JCAHO=With requirements for improvement. **Accreditation with the American Accreditation HealthCare Commission is shown as: AAHC. None=No accreditation action reported by any of the three accrediting organizations.**

Plan Ratings

✓ means plan receives our top rating
Highest scores are in **Blue**
Lowest scores are in ***Bold Italic***
"—" means no data

Footnotes are on page 56

	Doctors' overall rating of plan for patient care (% favorable)	Members' overall rating of plan (% favorable)	Direct measures of actual care for which plan was among the best or worst plans (see codes below)*		Accreditation status**	% of members who had a problem (lower is better)	
			Best	Worst or not reported		"Big" problem getting referrals/tests/care	Called/wrote plan with complaint or problem
Average for all plans	57	60				9	20
Illinois (continued)							
✓ John Deere Health Plan (HMO) (Central and northwestern Illinois)	—	72	defghijk	None	Excellent	5	14
Medical Associates Health Plans (Jo Daviess County)	—	69	d	abcghij	Commendable	—	—
Mercy Health Plans (HMO) (St. Louis area)	70	66	None	acdefghi	None	7	14
One Health Plan of Illinois (Chicago area)	65	—	—	—	None	—	—
OSF HealthCare (Northeastern Illinois)	—	65	ak	h	Accredited	9	20
✓ PersonalCare (HMO) (East-central Illinois)	—	67	adefghijk	None	Excellent	9	18
✓ Premier Plus by Mercy Health Plans (HMO) (St. Louis area)	—	75	—	—	None	5	9
UNICARE Health Plans of the Midwest (HMO) (Chicago area)	—	*47*	a	c	Commendable	*15*	*25*
✓ UnitedHealthcare of the Midwest (Southern Illinois)	75	69	None	bfghi	JCAHO	2	14
Indiana							
Aetna U.S. Healthcare (Indianapolis area)	56	*54*	d	i	Commendable	7	*32*
Aetna U.S. Healthcare (Northwestern Indiana)	*43*	*46*	None	bcdeghik	Commendable	*11*	*29*
Aetna U.S. Healthcare (Southern Indiana)	—	*45*	None	aci	None	*12*	*29*
Anthem Blue Cross and Blue Shield (Most of Indiana)	58	55	j	bcik	None	9	*31*
✓ Arnett Health Plans (North-central Indiana)	—	73	begjk	None	Excellent	6	14
BlueChoice (POS) (Northwestern Indiana)	—	55	None	bcefghj	Commendable	10	*29*
CIGNA HealthCare of Illinois (Northwestern Indiana)	58	55	ah	d	Commendable	*12*	23
CIGNA HealthCare of Indiana (Northern and central Indiana)	—	*51*	None	abgik	Commendable	*12*	*31*
HMO Illinois/BlueAdvantage (HMO) (Northwestern Indiana)	58	56	a	bchj	Excellent	*11*	23
Humana Health Plan–Illinois (HMO) (Northwestern Indiana)	*45*	*54*	a	bcegik	Commendable	*11*	23
Humana Health Plans (Southern Indiana)	—	60	h	dgk	None	10	*27*
Humana/ChoiceCare (Southeastern Indiana)	61	69	fj	None	Commendable	6	19
M•Plan (HMO) (Northeastern and central Indiana)	61	64	hi	a	Excellent	8	22
PARTNERS National Health Plans of Indiana (Northern Indiana)	—	68	j	bfg	None	8	17
UNICARE Health Plans of the Midwest (HMO) (Northwestern Indiana)	—	*47*	a	c	Commendable	*15*	*25*
UnitedHealthcare of Kentucky (Southern Indiana)	—	63	—	—	Excellent	6	18
✓ UnitedHealthcare of Ohio (Dearborn County)	61	62	ef	None	Excellent	5	23
Welborn Health Plans (Southwestern Indiana)	—	72	bdgik	a	Denied	5	18
Iowa							
Community Health Plan (Southwestern Iowa)	70	63	None	bdeijk	None	8	19
Coventry Health Care of Iowa (Central Iowa)	—	56	—	—	None	4	*16*
Exclusive Healthcare (Western Iowa)	—	—	bek	None	Excellent	—	—

*Assuring proper prevention and screening: a=Adolescent immunizations; b=Childhood immunizations; c=Chlamydia screening in sexually active women; d=Breast cancer screening; e=Cervical cancer screening. Assuring proper treatment: f=Beta blocker treatment after a heart attack; g=Cholesterol management (two measures); h=Controlling high blood pressure; i=Comprehensive diabetes care (six measures); j=Use of appropriate asthma medication; k=Followup after hospitalization for mental illness. "Best" or "worst" indicates plan's scores were in either the top or bottom 25 percent of benchmark plans.

Detailed performance measures

Ratings by doctors (% favorable)										Ratings by members (% favorable)									
Ability of patients to see appropriate specialists	Ability of patients to get needed tests and treatments	Ability of patients to get appropriate drugs	Plan's programs to help doctors give better care	How plan helps doctors follow up with patients	Incentives plan gives doctors affecting quality of care	Quality of primary care physicians affiliated with plan	Quality of specialists affiliated with plan	Quality of hospitals doctors can refer to within the plan	Number of doctors rating plan on the survey	Overall health care	Personal doctors	Specialist doctors	No problem getting referrals/tests/care	Getting care quickly	How well doctors communicate	Plan's customer service	Plan's claims processing	Estimated cost index for single person	Plan's phone number
56	56	52	42	36	30	72	76	78		73	75	77	79	78	90	67	81	$1.00	800-999-9999
–	–	–	–	–	–	–	–	–	–	81	79	81	89	86	93	72	92	–	800-224-6599
–	–	–	–	–	–	–	–	–	–	74	78	77	–	84	91	74	91	–	800-747-8900
61	61	57	29	24	26	87	85	82	40	79	74	85	83	82	91	73	91	$1.08	800-327-0763
61	64	61	39	45	35	71	74	75	66	–	–	–	–	–	–	–	–	–	800-663-8081
–	–	–	–	–	–	–	–	–	–	77	76	77	80	85	93	70	86	$0.96	309-655-2850
–	–	–	–	–	–	–	–	–	–	72	76	73	83	84	90	73	91	$0.78	800-431-1211
–	–	–	–	–	–	–	–	–	–	81	83	80	81	75	94	76	87	$1.02	800-280-1602
–	–	–	–	–	–	–	–	–	–	63	70	73	72	74	88	61	62	$0.72	312-234-7000
76	74	69	57	48	33	93	95	95	64	82	78	84	88	82	93	68	89	–	800-627-0687
51	53	51	40	35	30	80	79	83	223	75	77	79	80	82	92	63	76	$1.13[6]	800-323-9930
43	40	42	31	30	26	70	76	70	192	64	72	69	76	76	89	65	63	–	800-323-9930
–	–	–	–	–	–	–	–	–	–	74	76	70	75	78	90	60	68	$0.98	800-323-9930
46	50	51	26	23	14	76	76	74	36	71	73	77	79	84	91	58	79	–	317-488-6000
–	–	–	–	–	–	–	–	–	–	80	75	78	87	84	93	76	90	$1.02	765-448-7440
–	–	–	–	–	–	–	–	–	–	73	75	75	76	78	90	60	75	–	800-654-7385
55	52	48	41	37	33	76	78	77	158	66	68	66	75	77	88	65	80	–	800-832-3211
–	–	–	–	–	–	–	–	–	–	75	73	77	77	84	92	57	77	–	800-832-3211
54	54	55	46	39	35	74	76	76	189	68	71	66	76	76	88	62	70	–	800-892-2803
40	43	37	31	28	30	66	73	74	154	66	71	73	78	75	87	65	65	–	800-448-6262
–	–	–	–	–	–	–	–	–	–	73	76	78	78	77	90	64	79	$0.96	800-448-6262
53	57	53	33	38	22	78	79	82	87	70	68	75	85	79	90	75	88	–	800-448-6262
50	57	39	34	36	21	71	62	74	36	72	73	77	81	80	91	69	81	$1.12	800-816-7526
–	–	–	–	–	–	–	–	–	–	80	77	79	83	86	93	73	90	–	800-967-5439
–	–	–	–	–	–	–	–	–	–	63	70	73	72	74	88	61	62	$0.72	312-234-7000
–	–	–	–	–	–	–	–	–	–	78	81	78	88	80	90	69	80	–	502-326-3033
63	59	64	38	29	24	80	76	76	59	77	78	77	88	82	91	68	81	$1.21	800-231-2198
–	–	–	–	–	–	–	–	–	–	79	78	80	83	87	90	69	88	$1.09	800-521-0265
60	62	68	57	49	43	79	85	83	43	75	78	82	80	82	91	71	85	–	816-271-1247
–	–	–	–	–	–	–	–	–	–	77	76	75	85	84	92	61	84	$0.97	800-257-4692
–	–	–	–	–	–	–	–	–	–	–	–	–	–	–	–	–	–	–	800-631-4333

**Accreditation status with NCQA (1/2002) is shown. Accreditation status with JCAHO (1/2002) is shown as follows: JCAHO=With commendation or with full standards compliance; JCAHO=With requirements for improvement. Accreditation with the American Accreditation HealthCare Commission is shown as: AAHC. None=No accreditation action reported by any of the three accrediting organizations.

Plan Ratings

✓ means plan receives our top rating
Highest scores are in Blue
Lowest scores are in *Bold Italic*
"—" means no data

Footnotes are on page 56

	Doctors' overall rating of plan for patient care (% favorable)	Members' overall rating of plan (% favorable)	Direct measures of actual care for which plan was among the best or worst plans (see codes below)* Best	Worst or not reported	Accreditation status**	"Big" problem getting referrals/tests/care	Called/wrote plan with complaint or problem
Average for all plans	▇ 57	60				9	20
Iowa *(continued)*							
✓ Health Alliance (Eastern Iowa)	–	67	dhj	f	Excellent	8	*16*
✓ John Deere Health Plan (HMO) (Central and southeastern Iowa)	–	72	defghijk	None	Excellent	5	*14*
Medical Associates Health Plans (Northeastern Iowa)	–	69	d	abcghij	Commendable	–	–
Sioux Valley Health Plan (HMO) (Northwestern Iowa)	–	*48*	k	abj	JCAHO	6	22
✓ UnitedHealthcare of the Midlands (Western Iowa)	–	65	k	i	Excellent	5	20
Wellmark Health Plan of Iowa (Central Iowa)	–	58	deghi	fj	Excellent	9	23
Kansas							
Aetna U.S. Healthcare (Kansas City area)	▇ 66	*53*	None	acdhj	None	9	21
Blue Cross Blue Shield of Kansas (HMO) (Most of Kansas)	–	64	dj	a	None	6	17
Blue Cross Blue Shield of Kansas (POS) (Most of Kansas)	–	58	j	abf	None	6	19
BCBS of Kansas City/Blue-Advantage (HMO) (Kansas City area)	▇ 87	*53*	None	abdghij	AAHC	9	20
✓ BCBS of Kansas City/Blue-Care (HMO) (Kansas City area)	▇ 87	63	None	aceghi	AAHC	6	22
CIGNA HealthCare of Kansas/Missouri (Kansas City area)	▇ 51	*51*	None	None	Commendable	*12*	*27*
Community Health Plan (Northeastern Kansas)	▇ 70	63	None	bdeijk	None	8	19
Coventry Health Care of Kansas (Kansas City area)	▇ 62	56	None	bcfghjk	None	8	18
FirstGuard Health Plan (Most or all of Kansas)	▇ 75	60	–	–	None	6	*27*
Humana Health Plans (HMO) (Kansas City area)	▇ *42*	57	b	c	Commendable	*12*	23
Mid America Health[7] (HMO) (Kansas City area)	▇ 70	62	dejk	ah	None	8	21
Mid America Health[7] (POS) (Kansas City area)	▇ 70	62	ej	ach	None	5	20
✓ UnitedHealthcare of the Midwest (Eastern Kansas)	▇ 81	69	None	bfghi	JCAHO	2	22
Kentucky							
Aetna U.S. Healthcare (Lexington and Louisville areas)	–	*45*	None	aci	None	*12*	*29*
Aetna U.S. Healthcare (Northern Kentucky)	▇ 56	*54*	d	i	Commendable	7	*32*
Anthem Blue Cross & Blue Shield (Central, eastern, and northern KY)	–	68	hj	ak	None	5	20
✓ Bluegrass Family Health (Most of Kentucky)	–	68	–	–	None	4	*12*
CHA Health (Most of Kentucky)	–	61	fh	acijk	None	8	20
CIGNA HealthCare Ohio (Northern Kentucky)	▇ 56	55	None	None	Excellent	10	*30*
Humana Health Plans (Louisville area)	–	60	h	dgk	None	10	*27*
Humana/ChoiceCare (Northern Kentucky)	▇ 61	69	fj	None	Commendable	6	19
UnitedHealthcare of Kentucky (Most of Kentucky)	–	63	–	–	Excellent	6	18
✓ UnitedHealthcare of Ohio (Northern Kentucky)	▇ 61	62	ef	None	Excellent	5	23

*Assuring proper prevention and screening: a=Adolescent immunizations; b=Childhood immunizations; c=Chlamydia screening in sexually active women; d=Breast cancer screening; e=Cervical cancer screening. Assuring proper treatment: f=Beta blocker treatment after a heart attack; g=Cholesterol management (two measures); h=Controlling high blood pressure; i=Comprehensive diabetes care (six measures); j=Use of appropriate asthma medication; k=Followup after hospitalization for mental illness. "Best" or "worst" indicates plan's scores were in either the top or bottom 25 percent of benchmark plans.**

Detailed performance measures

Ratings by doctors (% favorable)										Ratings by members (% favorable)									
Ability of patients to see appropriate specialists	Ability of patients to get needed tests and treatments	Ability of patients to get appropriate drugs	Plan's programs to help doctors give better care	How plan helps doctors follow up with patients	Incentives plan gives doctors affecting quality of care	Quality of primary care physicians affiliated with plan	Quality of specialists affiliated with plan	Quality of hospitals doctors can refer to within the plan	Number of doctors rating plan on the survey	Overall health care	Personal doctors	Specialist doctors	No problem getting referrals/tests/care	Getting care quickly	How well doctors communicate	Plan's customer service	Plan's claims processing	Estimated cost index for single person	Plan's phone number
56	56	52	42	36	30	72	76	78		73	75	77	79	78	90	67	81	$1.00	800-999-9999
–	–	–	–	–	–	–	–	–	–	77	79	78	83	85	92	70	87	$1.13	800-851-3379
–	–	–	–	–	–	–	–	–	–	81	79	81	89	86	93	72	92	–	800-224-6599
–	–	–	–	–	–	–	–	–	–	74	78	77	–	84	91	74	91	–	800-747-8900
–	–	–	–	–	–	–	–	–	–	76	78	82	88	84	93	62	82	–	605-333-1000
–	–	–	–	–	–	–	–	–	–	79	78	79	89	87	92	70	88	–	800-284-0626
–	–	–	–	–	–	–	–	–	–	75	76	71	81	84	93	64	84	–	800-526-8995
64	59	60	45	44	31	75	76	71	87	71	72	76	79	77	90	67	78	–	800-323-9930
–	–	–	–	–	–	–	–	–	–	72	75	72	86	84	93	71	93	–	800-874-1823
–	–	–	–	–	–	–	–	–	–	74	73	72	86	84	93	65	92	–	800-874-1823
81	83	76	62	67	51	94	94	93	92	66	71	75	79	76	88	63	83	–	816-395-2222
81	83	76	62	67	51	94	94	93	92	73	77	79	85	79	90	64	86	–	816-395-2222
57	54	45	43	42	33	71	72	69	69	66	66	73	74	77	87	54	76	–	800-832-3211
60	62	68	57	49	43	79	85	83	43	75	78	82	80	82	91	71	85	–	816-271-1247
60	55	50	48	43	35	73	78	73	87	79	74	77	82	80	91	62	86	–	800-969-3343
73	75	73	59	51	38	84	82	80	55	70	73	75	81	78	89	70	73	–	888-828-5698
31	43	40	35	35	26	56	65	62	60	65	73	72	77	77	87	62	74	$0.91	800-448-6262
71	68	68	57	51	42	81	83	79	96	71	76	80	81	78	91	64	81	–	800-632-4765
71	68	68	57	51	42	81	83	79	96	76	79	77	90	82	90	63	81	–	800-632-4765
73	73	78	64	58	54	86	90	85	73	75	74	77	89	80	91	67	85	–	800-627-0687
–	–	–	–	–	–	–	–	–	–	74	76	70	75	78	90	60	68	$0.98	800-323-9930
51	53	51	40	35	30	80	79	83	223	75	77	79	80	82	92	63	76	$1.13[6]	800-323-9930
–	–	–	–	–	–	–	–	–	–	76	75	82	85	81	91	73	87	–	502-423-2011
–	–	–	–	–	–	–	–	–	–	81	78	83	84	83	94	74	93	–	800-787-2680
–	–	–	–	–	–	–	–	–	–	78	76	79	81	79	92	70	87	–	800-457-5683
54	53	52	40	33	30	81	83	83	171	73	72	76	76	80	91	64	80	–	800-832-3211
–	–	–	–	–	–	–	–	–	–	73	76	78	78	77	90	64	79	$0.96	800-448-6262
53	57	53	33	38	22	78	79	82	87	70	68	75	85	79	90	75	88	–	800-448-6262
–	–	–	–	–	–	–	–	–	–	78	81	78	88	80	90	69	80	–	502-326-3033
63	59	64	38	29	24	80	76	76	59	77	78	77	88	82	91	68	81	$1.21	800-231-2198

Accreditation status with NCQA (1/2002) is shown. Accreditation status with JCAHO (1/2002) is shown as follows: JCAHO=With commendation or with full standards compliance; JCAHO=With requirements for improvement. **Accreditation with the American **Accreditation HealthCare Commission is shown as: AAHC. None=No accreditation action** reported by any of the three accrediting organizations.

Plan Ratings

✓ means plan receives our top rating
Highest scores are in Blue
Lowest scores are in *Bold Italic*
"–" means no data

Footnotes are on page 56

	Doctors' overall rating of plan for patient care (% favorable)	Members' overall rating of plan (% favorable)	Key performance measures — Direct measures of actual care for which plan was among the best or worst plans (see codes below)* — Best	Worst or not reported	Accreditation status**	% of members who had a problem (lower is better) — "Big" problem getting referrals/tests/care	Called/wrote plan with complaint or problem
Average for all plans	57	60				9	20
Louisiana							
Aetna U.S. Healthcare (Southeastern Louisiana)	68	61	–	–	None	5	21
CIGNA HealthCare of Louisiana (Southeastern Louisiana)	70	–	–	–	None	–	–
The OATH for Louisiana (All of Louisiana)	67	–	–	–	None	–	–
Ochsner Health Plan (HMO) (Southeastern Louisiana)	–	60	bg	fjk	In process	*12*	24
UnitedHealthcare of Louisiana (All or most of Louisiana)	75	–	–	–	JCAHO	–	–
Maine							
Aetna U.S. Healthcare (All or most of Maine)	–	57	defhik	bcj	Excellent	5	20
✓ Anthem Blue Cross and Blue Shield (All or most of Maine)	–	57	defgik	None	Excellent	7	21
CIGNA HealthCare of Maine (Most of Maine)	–	61	acdefgik	b	Excellent	8	22
✓ Harvard Pilgrim Health Care (All or most of Maine)	72	67	abcdejk	None	Commendable	7	13
HMO New England (All or most of Maine)	50	–	–	–	None	–	–
Maine Partners Health Plan[2] (Southwestern Maine)	–	57	degi	None	None	5	18
Maryland							
Aetna U.S. Healthcare (Eastern and central Maryland)	*39*	*48*	bfh	cg	Commendable	*12*	23
AmeriHealth HMO of Delaware (Eastern Maryland)	51	59	a	cehj	Excellent	8	*24*
Capital Care/CareFirst (Washington area)	63	58	bdj	h	Excellent	9	23
CIGNA HealthCare Mid-Atlantic (Central Maryland)	50	*48*	bch	i	Excellent	*13*	22
Coventry Health Care (Most of Maryland)	*36*	63	acd	gjk	None	6	*28*
Delmarva Health Plan (Eastern shore)	–	70	None	ghj	None	5	17
Free State Health Plan (All of Maryland)	*38*	57	b	chk	Excellent	9	18
Kaiser Foundation HP Mid-Atlantic States (HMO) (Central MD)	56	60	abcef	None	Commendable	10	13
M.D. IPA (All of Maryland)	50	70	bhj	f	Excellent	7	20
Optimum Choice (All of Maryland)	54	62	b	f	Excellent	9	16
Preferred Health Network[2] (Eastern and central Maryland)	70	*51*	–	–	None	6	*29*
UnitedHealthcare of the Mid-Atlantic (HMO) (All or most of Maryland)	57	*54*	–	–	JCAHO	5	25
Massachusetts							
Aetna U.S. Healthcare (All or most of Massachusetts)	*44*	*52*	abh	None	Commendable	9	*24*
✓ BlueCHiP (Southeastern Massachusetts)	57	67	eh	fij	Excellent	6	17
✓ BlueCross BlueShield of MA/HMO Blue (All or most of MA)	84	74	abdefk	None	Excellent	4	15
CIGNA HealthCare of Massachusetts (Most of Massachusetts)	55	62	abcdegh	None	Excellent	8	*27*
✓ ConnectiCare (Southwestern Massachusetts)	60	68	bcdefjk	h	Excellent	7	16
Fallon Community Health Plan (Eastern and central Massachusetts)	*37*	66	acdefghk	None	Excellent	7	15

*Assuring proper prevention and screening: a=Adolescent immunizations; b=Childhood immunizations; c=Chlamydia screening in sexually active women; d=Breast cancer screening; e=Cervical cancer screening. **Assuring proper treatment:** f=Beta blocker treatment after a heart attack; g=Cholesterol management (two measures); h=Controlling high blood pressure; i=Comprehensive diabetes care (six measures); j=Use of appropriate asthma medication; k=Followup after hospitalization for mental illness. "Best" or "worst" indicates plan's scores were in either the top or bottom 25 percent of benchmark plans.

Detailed performance measures

Ratings by doctors (% favorable)										Ratings by members (% favorable)									
Ability of patients to see appropriate specialists	Ability of patients to get needed tests and treatments	Ability of patients to get appropriate drugs	Plan's programs to help doctors give better care	How plan helps doctors follow up with patients	Incentives plan gives doctors affecting quality of care	Quality of primary care physicians affiliated with plan	Quality of specialists affiliated with plan	Quality of hospitals doctors can refer to within the plan	Number of doctors rating plan on the survey	Overall health care	Personal doctors	Specialist doctors	No problem getting referrals/tests/care	Getting care quickly	How well doctors communicate	Plan's customer service	Plan's claims processing	Estimated cost index for single person	Plan's phone number
56	56	52	42	36	30	72	76	78		73	75	77	79	78	90	67	81	$1.00	800-999-9999
68	63	71	58	60	36	89	87	89	37	74	75	79	78	76	91	67	78	—	800-323-9930
71	71	70	55	62	40	83	80	76	27	—	—	—	—	—	—	—	—	—	800-832-3211
69	63	68	52	54	30	85	85	88	33	—	—	—	—	—	—	—	—	—	800-259-7370
—	—	—	—	—	—	—	—	—	—	70	78	75	71	72	89	66	77	—	800-701-2080
76	76	79	68	63	46	89	91	94	36	—	—	—	—	—	—	—	—	—	800-349-1000
—	—	—	—	—	—	—	—	—	—	79	78	81	86	87	93	69	83	—	800-323-9930
—	—	—	—	—	—	—	—	—	—	76	71	82	85	85	93	70	87	—	800-482-0966
—	—	—	—	—	—	—	—	—	—	77	72	80	82	85	92	65	89	—	800-832-3211
70	73	62	55	47	43	85	87	89	261	72	73	77	84	80	89	73	88	—	888-888-4742
51	61	52	40	26	21	80	81	79	30	—	—	—	—	—	—	—	—	—	800-331-0150
—	—	—	—	—	—	—	—	—	—	79	74	83	86	85	94	76	82	—	800-482-0966
39	38	41	29	20	18	62	66	75	351	68	71	74	76	76	89	60	74	$1.08	800-323-9930
48	49	41	34	30	22	76	79	78	155	73	73	72	82	82	91	65	78	—	302-777-6400
62	62	59	44	37	33	78	81	82	305	71	72	77	80	77	87	65	80	$1.02	800-296-5555
50	50	45	31	28	21	65	68	72	254	64	68	72	74	76	88	65	76	—	800-832-3211
42	37	40	30	14	18	66	69	70	47	75	72	78	87	82	90	65	77	—	800-833-7423
—	—	—	—	—	—	—	—	—	—	78	79	83	90	81	93	76	89	—	800-334-3427
36	36	39	26	20	18	50	51	58	128	67	76	77	81	77	89	67	82	—	800-445-6036
53	52	64	55	48	46	60	64	77	179	63	73	64	78	77	85	74	64	$0.86	800-777-7902
50	49	51	34	31	25	69	73	73	319	73	71	75	84	78	90	75	87	$0.96	800-782-1966
54	51	52	37	32	26	72	76	76	314	69	68	77	79	75	88	70	83	—	800-331-2102
69	66	58	38	32	32	74	79	80	135	72	77	78	81	75	91	55	69	—	800-422-1996
63	60	49	35	29	25	67	73	78	223	73	78	77	84	77	89	57	71	—	800-368-1680
43	50	45	33	28	25	67	71	75	248	74	76	80	79	80	91	60	70	—	800-323-9930
59	62	47	37	29	24	83	88	86	150	81	80	82	85	84	93	71	84	$1.07	401-274-3500
79	83	70	62	53	53	89	93	94	247	76	74	79	89	83	92	76	90	—	800-262-2583
55	63	58	41	37	36	76	80	78	173	76	77	79	83	83	93	63	76	—	800-832-3211
64	59	50	45	36	24	82	81	82	170	79	77	80	86	84	93	75	90	$0.94	800-251-7722
33	42	37	31	30	26	61	59	62	85	73	78	73	84	82	93	80	84	$1.09	800-868-5200

Accreditation status with NCQA (1/2002) is shown. Accreditation status with JCAHO (1/2002) is shown as follows: JCAHO=With commendation or with full standards compliance; JCAHO=With requirements for improvement. **Accreditation with the American

Accreditation HealthCare Commission is shown as: AAHC. None=No accreditation action reported by any of the three accrediting organizations.

Plan Ratings

✓ means plan receives our top rating
Highest scores are in Blue
Lowest scores are in *Bold Italic*
"—" means no data

Footnotes are on page 56

	Doctors' overall rating of plan for patient care (% favorable)	Members' overall rating of plan (% favorable)	Direct measures of actual care for which plan was among the best or worst plans (see codes below)*		Accreditation status**	% of members who had a problem (lower is better)	
			Best	Worst or not reported		"Big" problem getting referrals/tests/care	Called/wrote plan with complaint or problem
Average for all plans	57	60				9	20
Massachusetts (*continued*)							
✓ Harvard Pilgrim Health Care (All or most of Massachusetts)	72	67	abcdejk	None	Commendable	7	13
✓ Health New England (Western Massachusetts)	–	73	acfk	hi	Excellent	5	12
HMO New England (All or most of Massachusetts)	50	–	–	–	None	–	–
Neighborhood Health Plan (HMO) (Eastern Massachusetts)	59	68	abceh	None	None	10	20
One Health Plan of Massachusetts (Most of Massachusetts)	49	–	–	–	None	–	–
✓ Tufts Health Plan (HMO) (All or most of Massachusetts)	72	65	abcdefk	ghi	Excellent	8	15
✓ Tufts Health Plan (POS) (All or most of Massachusetts)	72	67	abcdfjk	ghi	Excellent	6	16
✓ UnitedHealthcare of New England (Southeastern and central MA)	57	71	abck	None	Excellent	5	18
Michigan							
Aetna U.S. Healthcare (Detroit area)	73	–	–	–	None	–	–
Blue Care Network of Michigan (HMO) (All or most of Michigan)	54	59	chk	g	Excellent[8]	10	20
Blue Cross Blue Shield of Michigan (POS) (All or most of Michigan)	–	61	ehk	gj	AAHC	8	22
✓ Care Choices (HMO) (Central Michigan)	63	64	bdijk	c	Excellent	8	17
CIGNA HealthCare of Indiana (Southwestern Michigan)	–	*51*	None	abgik	Commendable	*12*	*31*
✓ Grand Valley Health Plan (HMO) (Grand Rapids area)	–	68	cdei	abhj	Excellent	9	13
✓ HAP (HMO) (Southeastern Michigan)	70	68	abcdfhjk	None	Excellent	8	13
✓ HealthPlus of Michigan (Central Michigan)	*42*	81	cdefhk	None	Excellent	6	12
✓ M-CARE (HMO) (Southeastern Michigan)	75	65	defhijk	None	Excellent	11	13
OmniCare Health Plan[2] (HMO) (Southeastern Michigan)	*19*	*52*	None	abcdeghijk	Provisional	*13*	*28*
OmniCare Health Plan[2] (POS) (Southeastern Michigan)	*19*	*52*	None	abcdeghij	Provisional	*15*	*30*
✓ Paramount Health Care (HMO) (Southeastern Michigan)	–	73	e	ghj	Commendable	5	15
✓ Physicians Health Plan of Mid-Michigan (Central Michigan)	–	74	dejk	cgh	Excellent	6	18
Physicians Health Plan of South Michigan (South-central Michigan)	–	69	dk	ghi	JCAHO	6	19
Physicians Health Plan of Southwest Michigan (Southwestern MI)	–	59	bj	ah	JCAHO	7	*27*
✓ Priority Health (HMO) (Most of western Michigan)	–	72	deijk	c	Excellent	6	13
Total Health Care (Southeastern Michigan)	*26*	–	–	–	None	–	–
Ultimed HMO of Michigan (Detroit area)	*30*	–	–	–	None	–	–
The Wellness Plan (HMO) (Southeastern Michigan)	*22*	*50*	–	–	None	*13*	*28*
Minnesota							
✓ Blue Plus (All or most of Minnesota)	74	59	dj	None	Excellent	9	18
✓ HealthPartners Classic (Twin Cities area)	61	62	dg	i	Excellent	9	14
✓ Medica (Most of Minnesota)	72	64	None	g	Excellent	8	15

*Assuring proper prevention and screening: a=Adolescent immunizations; b=Childhood immunizations; c=Chlamydia screening in sexually active women; d=Breast cancer screening; e=Cervical cancer screening. Assuring proper treatment: f=Beta blocker treatment after a heart attack; g=Cholesterol management (two measures); h=Controlling high blood pressure; i=Comprehensive diabetes care (six measures); j=Use of appropriate asthma medication; k=Followup after hospitalization for mental illness. "Best" or "worst" indicates plan's scores were in either the top or bottom 25 percent of benchmark plans.

Detailed performance measures

Ratings by doctors (% favorable)										Ratings by members (% favorable)									
Ability of patients to see appropriate specialists	Ability of patients to get needed tests and treatments	Ability of patients to get appropriate drugs	Plan's programs to help doctors give better care	How plan helps doctors follow up with patients	Incentives plan gives doctors affecting quality of care	Quality of primary care physicians affiliated with plan	Quality of specialists affiliated with plan	Quality of hospitals doctors can refer to within the plan	Number of doctors rating plan on the survey	Overall health care	Personal doctors	Specialist doctors	No problem getting referrals/tests/care	Getting care quickly	How well doctors communicate	Plan's customer service	Plan's claims processing	Estimated cost index for single person	Plan's phone number
56	56	52	42	36	30	72	76	78		73	75	77	79	78	90	67	81	$1.00	800-999-9999
70	73	62	55	47	43	85	87	89	261	72	73	77	84	80	89	73	88	–	888-888-4742
–	–	–	–	–	–	–	–	–	–	78	78	79	90	85	92	80	92	$1.11	800-842-4464
51	61	52	40	26	21	80	81	79	30	–	–	–	–	–	–	–	–	–	800-331-0150
62	69	52	44	36	42	72	78	77	113	73	79	69	77	74	89	72	69	–	800-433-5556
54	65	55	42	32	33	68	74	77	35	–	–	–	–	–	–	–	–	–	800-663-8081
70	75	62	57	48	44	86	87	90	335	78	73	81	83	81	92	75	85	–	800-462-0224
70	75	62	57	48	44	86	87	90	335	78	78	83	86	84	94	73	82	–	800-843-1008
60	65	49	44	35	27	80	82	84	261	80	80	80	89	84	92	73	89	–	800-447-1245
70	70	72	59	51	45	85	88	86	120	–	–	–	–	–	–	–	–	–	800-323-9930
48	52	52	44	35	32	73	81	80	167	74	76	76	78	80	90	63	80	$0.76[9]	800-662-6667
–	–	–	–	–	–	–	–	–	–	76	77	79	82	83	92	63	84	–	800-662-6667
53	57	54	48	39	36	75	82	77	92	78	76	78	83	83	93	70	83	–	800-852-9780
–	–	–	–	–	–	–	–	–	–	75	73	77	77	84	92	57	77	–	800-832-3211
–	–	–	–	–	–	–	–	–	–	74	75	81	82	89	90	83	88	$0.93	616-949-2410
60	62	60	61	52	43	81	89	86	177	71	74	76	82	77	89	72	82	$0.99	800-422-4641
44	48	43	35	38	38	57	55	64	26	83	76	88	87	82	93	82	93	$1.00	800-332-9161
65	65	70	59	53	45	83	89	84	125	71	73	77	77	78	90	72	85	$0.83	800-658-8878
25	22	24	20	13	13	34	46	46	70	63	68	74	71	64	85	62	61	$0.83	800-925-4550
25	22	24	20	13	13	34	46	46	70	66	71	81	70	68	86	59	53	–	800-925-4550
–	–	–	–	–	–	–	–	–	–	80	76	82	88	84	95	73	91	$1.07	800-462-3589
–	–	–	–	–	–	–	–	–	–	82	79	84	87	85	94	74	87	–	800-832-9186
–	–	–	–	–	–	–	–	–	–	77	75	78	83	85	91	71	87	–	800-394-7569
–	–	–	–	–	–	–	–	–	–	75	73	79	83	84	92	66	81	–	800-548-6574
–	–	–	–	–	–	–	–	–	–	81	82	80	87	86	93	74	92	–	800-446-5674
21	23	23	17	17	17	46	51	46	39	–	–	–	–	–	–	–	–	–	313-871-2000
32	34	33	30	31	25	49	65	64	33	–	–	–	–	–	–	–	–	–	800-242-7955
22	22	18	22	18	14	34	53	43	68	65	73	75	71	74	86	60	64	$0.75	800-875-WELL
68	72	68	48	35	34	86	92	90	185	73	77	76	83	81	91	65	85	–	800-382-2000
53	65	53	61	47	41	75	80	77	231	73	75	70	82	81	90	70	85	$1.14	800-883-2177
74	75	62	49	36	34	89	95	91	206	80	83	81	85	80	92	69	86	–	800-952-3455

Accreditation status with NCQA (1/2002) is shown. Accreditation status with JCAHO (1/2002) is shown as follows: JCAHO=With commendation or with full standards compliance; JCAHO=With requirements for improvement. **Accreditation with the American**

Accreditation HealthCare Commission is shown as: AAHC. None=No accreditation action reported by any of the three accrediting organizations.

Plan Ratings

✓ means plan receives our top rating

Highest scores are in Blue

Lowest scores are in *Bold Italic*

"—" means no data

Footnotes are on page 56

	Doctors' overall rating of plan for patient care (% favorable)	Members' overall rating of plan (% favorable)	Direct measures of actual care for which plan was among the best or worst plans (see codes below)* Best	Direct measures of actual care for which plan was among the best or worst plans (see codes below)* Worst or not reported	Accreditation status**	"Big" problem getting referrals/tests/care	Called/wrote plan with complaint or problem
Average for all plans	57	60				9	20
Minnesota (continued)							
PreferredOne (Most of Minnesota)	84	–	–	–	AAHC	–	–
Sioux Valley Health Plan (HMO) (Southwestern Minnesota)	–	*48*	k	abj	JCAHO	6	22
Sioux Valley Health Plan of Minnesota (HMO) (Southwestern MN)	–	*41*	d	cj	None	5	23
Mississippi							
Aetna U.S. Healthcare (Northwestern Mississippi)	–	59	None	abcdefghijk	Accredited	–	–
CIGNA HealthCare of Louisiana (Pearl River and Hancock counties)	70	–	–	–	None	–	–
Missouri							
Aetna U.S. Healthcare (Kansas City area)	66	*53*	None	acdhj	None	9	21
Aetna U.S. Healthcare (St. Louis area)	52	–	–	–	None	–	–
BCBS of Kansas City/Blue-Advantage (HMO) (Kansas City area)	87	*53*	None	abdghij	AAHC	9	20
✓ BCBS of Kansas City/Blue-Care (HMO) (Kansas City area)	87	63	None	aceghi	AAHC	6	22
BlueCHOICE (Eastern and southern Missouri)	*44*	57	None	cfgijk	Commendable	7	16
CIGNA HealthCare of Kansas/Missouri (Kansas City area)	51	*51*	None	None	Commendable	*12*	*27*
✓ CIGNA HealthCare of St. Louis (St. Louis area)	74	63	abfh	None	Commendable	8	18
Community Health Plan (Northwestern Missouri)	70	63	None	bdeijk	None	8	19
Coventry Health Care of Kansas (Kansas City area)	62	56	None	bcfghjk	None	8	18
Cox HealthPlans (Southwestern Missouri)	–	*52*	–	–	None	3	19
FirstGuard Health Plan (Kansas City area)	75	60	–	–	None	6	*27*
Group Health Plan (St. Louis area)	*38*	65	abj	ceik	None	9	16
✓ HealthLink (HMO) (Northeastern, east-central, and southwestern MO)	71	66	–	–	None	4	13
HealthLink (POS) (Northeastern, east-central, and southwestern MO)	71	65	–	–	None	6	20
Humana Health Plans (HMO) (Kansas City area)	*42*	57	b	c	Commendable	*12*	23
Mercy Health Plans (HMO) (Eastern and central Missouri)	70	66	None	acdefghi	None	7	14
Mid America Health[7] (HMO) (Kansas City area)	70	62	dejk	ah	None	8	21
Mid America Health[7] (POS) (Kansas City area)	70	62	ej	ach	None	5	20
Premier Health Plans (HMO) (Southwestern Missouri)	–	65	j	cfhik	None	7	15
✓ Premier Plus by Mercy Health Plans (HMO) (Eastern Missouri)	–	75	–	–	None	5	9
✓ UnitedHealthcare of the Midwest (Most of eastern Missouri)	75	69	None	bfghi	JCAHO	2	14
✓ UnitedHealthcare of the Midwest (Most of western Missouri)	81	69	None	bfghi	JCAHO	2	22
Nebraska							
Exclusive Healthcare (Eastern Nebraska)	–	–	bek	None	Excellent	–	–

*Assuring proper prevention and screening: a=Adolescent immunizations; b=Childhood immunizations; c=Chlamydia screening in sexually active women; d=Breast cancer screening; e=Cervical cancer screening. Assuring proper treatment: f=Beta blocker treatment after a heart attack; g=Cholesterol management (two measures); h=Controlling high blood pressure; i=Comprehensive diabetes care (six measures); j=Use of appropriate asthma medication; k=Followup after hospitalization for mental illness. "Best" or "worst" indicates plan's scores were in either the top or bottom 25 percent of benchmark plans.

Detailed performance measures

Ratings by doctors (% favorable)										Ratings by members (% favorable)									
Ability of patients to see appropriate specialists	Ability of patients to get needed tests and treatments	Ability of patients to get appropriate drugs	Plan's programs to help doctors give better care	How plan helps doctors follow up with patients	Incentives plan gives doctors affecting quality of care	Quality of primary care physicians affiliated with plan	Quality of specialists affiliated with plan	Quality of hospitals doctors can refer to within the plan	Number of doctors rating plan on the survey	Overall health care	Personal doctors	Specialist doctors	No problem getting referrals/tests/care	Getting care quickly	How well doctors communicate	Plan's customer service	Plan's claims processing	Estimated cost index for single person	Plan's phone number
56	56	52	42	36	30	72	76	78		73	75	77	79	78	90	67	81	$1.00	800-999-9999
86	82	79	48	36	36	90	93	94	180	–	–	–	–	–	–	–	–	–	800-379-7727
–	–	–	–	–	–	–	–	–	–	76	78	82	88	84	93	62	82	–	605-333-1000
–	–	–	–	–	–	–	–	–	–	83	81	84	88	89	95	61	87	–	605-333-1000
–	–	–	–	–	–	–	–	–	–	68	79	75	–	67	86	69	81	$0.90	800-323-9930
71	71	70	55	62	40	83	80	76	27	–	–	–	–	–	–	–	–	–	800-832-3211
64	59	60	45	44	31	75	76	71	87	71	72	76	79	77	90	67	78	–	800-323-9930
56	62	65	29	31	24	79	83	81	56	–	–	–	–	–	–	–	–	–	800-323-9930
81	83	76	62	67	51	94	94	93	92	66	71	75	79	76	88	63	83	–	816-395-2222
81	83	76	62	67	51	94	94	93	92	73	77	79	85	79	90	64	86	–	816-395-2222
52	52	57	33	24	28	74	85	80	52	74	76	76	84	81	92	64	86	$0.98	800-932-4480
57	54	45	43	42	33	71	72	69	69	66	66	73	74	77	87	54	76	–	800-832-3211
70	71	60	40	35	21	85	91	91	57	75	71	78	81	82	91	69	89	–	800-832-3211
60	62	68	57	49	43	79	85	83	43	75	78	82	80	82	91	71	85	–	816-271-1247
60	55	50	48	43	35	73	78	73	87	79	74	77	82	80	91	62	86	–	800-969-3343
–	–	–	–	–	–	–	–	–	–	74	77	77	85	79	92	63	88	–	800-664-1244
73	75	73	59	51	38	84	82	80	55	70	73	75	81	78	89	70	73	–	888-828-5698
41	39	36	32	22	17	65	82	81	68	81	75	81	81	81	91	69	87	$1.18	800-755-3901
69	74	73	38	35	26	81	83	86	63	80	76	85	84	80	91	67	89	–	800-624-2356
69	74	73	38	35	26	81	83	86	63	76	76	81	81	84	91	65	85	–	800-624-2356
31	43	40	35	35	26	56	65	62	60	65	73	72	77	77	87	62	74	$0.91	800-448-6262
61	61	57	29	24	26	87	85	82	40	79	74	85	83	82	91	73	91	$1.08	800-327-0763
71	68	68	57	51	42	81	83	79	96	71	76	80	81	78	91	64	81	–	800-632-4765
71	68	68	57	51	42	81	83	79	96	76	79	77	90	82	90	63	81	–	800-632-4765
–	–	–	–	–	–	–	–	–	–	79	72	81	84	82	92	67	88	$1.08	800-836-0402
–	–	–	–	–	–	–	–	–	–	81	83	80	81	75	94	76	87	$1.02	800-280-1602
76	74	69	57	48	33	93	95	95	64	82	78	84	88	82	93	68	89	–	800-627-0687
73	73	78	64	58	54	86	90	85	73	75	74	77	89	80	91	67	85	–	800-627-0687
–	–	–	–	–	–	–	–	–	–	–	–	–	–	–	–	–	–	–	800-631-4333

Accreditation status with NCQA (1/2002) is shown. Accreditation status with JCAHO (1/2002) is shown as follows: JCAHO=With commendation or with full standards compliance; JCAHO=With requirements for improvement. **Accreditation with the American **Accreditation HealthCare Commission is shown as: AAHC.** None=No accreditation action reported by any of the three accrediting organizations.

Plan Ratings

✓ means plan receives our top rating
Highest scores are in Blue
Lowest scores are in *Bold Italic*
"—" means no data

Footnotes are on page 56

	Key performance measures						
	Doctors' overall rating of plan for patient care (% favorable)	Members' overall rating of plan (% favorable)	Direct measures of actual care for which plan was among the best or worst plans (see codes below)*		Accreditation status**	% of members who had a problem (lower is better)	
			Best	Worst or not reported		"Big" problem getting referrals/tests/care	Called/wrote plan with complaint or problem
Average for all plans	57	60				9	20
Nebraska (continued)							
Sioux Valley Health Plan (HMO) (Northeastern Nebraska)	–	*48*	k	abj	JCAHO	6	22
✓ UnitedHealthcare of the Midlands (Eastern Nebraska)	–	65	k	i	Excellent	5	20
Nevada							
Aetna U.S. Healthcare (Southern Nevada)	47	*50*	c	abdjk	None	*12*	20
Health Plan of Nevada (Southern and western Nevada)	*19*	43	None	abcdeghijk	Accredited	–	–
HMO Nevada (All or most of Nevada)	*38*	–	–	–	None	–	–
NevadaCare (Las Vegas area)	*39*				None		
PacifiCare of Nevada (HMO) (Southern and western Nevada)	*36*	52	None	abcdeghj	Commendable	*14*	23
New Hampshire							
✓ Anthem Blue Cross and Blue Shield (All or most of New Hampshire)	–	57	bdefgijk	None	Excellent	7	17
✓ BlueCross BlueShield of MA/HMO Blue (Southeastern NH)	84	74	abdefk	None	Excellent	4	*15*
✓ CIGNA HealthCare of New Hampshire (All of New Hampshire)		64	cdefgijk	None	Excellent	9	19
✓ Harvard Pilgrim Health Care of New England (Most of NH)	–	65	bdjk	None	Commendable	7	18
HMO New England (All or most of New Hampshire)	50	–	–	–	None	–	–
✓ Tufts Health Plan (HMO) (Southern New Hampshire)	72	65	abcdefk	ghi	Excellent	8	*15*
✓ Tufts Health Plan (POS) (Southern New Hampshire)	72	67	abcdfjk	ghi	Excellent	6	16
New Jersey							
Aetna U.S. Healthcare (Northern New Jersey)	*32*	56	None	cdh	Excellent	8	16
✓ Aetna U.S. Healthcare (Southern New Jersey)	56	68	bi	None	Excellent	5	14
AmeriHealth HMO of New Jersey (All of New Jersey)	*43*	58	bf	j	Excellent	7	*26*
CIGNA HealthCare of New Jersey (All of New Jersey)	51	*54*	None	cdhi	Commendable	7	*27*
Coventry Health Care (Southwestern New Jersey)	*36*	63	acd	gjk	None	6	*28*
Health Net of the Northeast[1] (All of New Jersey)	60	63	–	–	None	5	22
Horizon HMO (HMO) (All of New Jersey)	54	*54*	None	defj	Commendable	10	*30*
Keystone Health Plan East (All or most of New Jersey)	*40*	65	abi	cde	Excellent	8	13
One Health Plan (All or most of New Jersey)	55	*46*	–	–	None	8	*35*
Oxford Health Plans (All or most of New Jersey)	51	58	fgj	None	Commendable	8	18
UnitedHealthcare of New Jersey (All or most of New Jersey)	63	55	None	cdehi	Commendable	8	*29*
University Health Plans (All of New Jersey)	*43*	–	–	–	None	–	–
WellChoice HMO of New Jersey[10] (Northern New Jersey)	–	56	–	–	None	5	*30*

*Assuring proper prevention and screening: a=Adolescent immunizations; b=Childhood immunizations; c=Chlamydia screening in sexually active women; d=Breast cancer screening; e=Cervical cancer screening. **Assuring proper treatment:** f=Beta blocker treatment after a heart attack; g=Cholesterol management (two measures); h=Controlling high blood pressure; i=Comprehensive diabetes care (six measures); j=Use of appropriate asthma medication; k=Followup after hospitalization for mental illness. "Best" or "worst" indicates plan's scores were in either the top or bottom 25 percent of benchmark plans.

Detailed performance measures

Ratings by doctors (% favorable)										Ratings by members (% favorable)									
Ability of patients to see appropriate specialists	Ability of patients to get needed tests and treatments	Ability of patients to get appropriate drugs	Plan's programs to help doctors give better care	How plan helps doctors follow up with patients	Incentives plan gives doctors affecting quality of care	Quality of primary care physicians affiliated with plan	Quality of specialists affiliated with plan	Quality of hospitals doctors can refer to within the plan	Number of doctors rating plan on the survey	Overall health care	Personal doctors	Specialist doctors	No problem getting referrals/tests/care	Getting care quickly	How well doctors communicate	Plan's customer service	Plan's claims processing	Estimated cost index for single person	Plan's phone number
56	56	52	42	36	30	72	76	78		73	75	77	79	78	90	67	81	$1.00	800-999-9999
–	–	–	–	–	–	–	–	–	–	76	78	82	88	84	93	62	82	–	605-333-1000
–	–	–	–	–	–	–	–	–	–	79	78	79	89	87	92	70	88	–	800-284-0626
55	52	49	37	33	25	73	71	72	62	61	67	75	73	69	81	68	74	$0.95	800-323-9930
23	16	21	21	16	13	27	44	62	57	53	69	59	–	66	82	55	77	$0.84	800-777-1840
37	41	44	38	32	28	67	63	70	42	–	–	–	–	–	–	–	–	–	800-438-5270
42	40	35	33	32	25	59	65	71	61	–	–	–	–	–	–	–	–	–	702-304-5500
37	37	26	29	33	21	43	43	58	42	61	63	72	71	68	83	65	81	$0.94	800-826-4347
–	–	–	–	–	–	–	–	–	–	75	73	76	83	84	91	70	87	–	800-438-9672
79	83	70	62	53	53	89	93	94	247	76	74	79	89	83	92	76	90	–	800-262-2583
–	–	–	–	–	–	–	–	–	–	75	74	78	81	84	91	69	90	–	800-832-3211
–	–	–	–	–	–	–	–	–	–	74	73	74	84	85	92	71	88	–	888-888-4742
51	61	52	40	26	21	80	81	79	30	–	–	–	–	–	–	–	–	–	800-331-0150
70	75	62	57	48	44	86	87	90	335	78	73	81	83	81	92	75	85	–	800-462-0224
70	75	62	57	48	44	86	87	90	335	78	78	83	86	84	94	73	82	–	800-843-1008
31	32	36	25	20	18	58	58	65	320	70	75	74	82	78	91	64	79	$1.17	800-323-9930
58	55	41	39	33	25	80	89	86	124	77	82	82	87	82	93	72	86	$1.17	800-323-9930
43	42	40	30	27	21	64	64	70	403	73	76	77	83	82	91	67	77	$1.08	856-778-6500
52	49	42	36	33	27	75	75	79	346	68	70	74	75	76	90	62	73	–	800-832-3211
42	37	40	30	14	18	66	69	70	47	75	72	78	87	82	90	65	77	–	800-833-7423
62	58	56	40	35	31	75	73	77	545	74	76	77	83	78	91	67	76	$1.35	800-909-3447
57	54	54	38	33	29	75	73	78	348	70	72	74	79	76	89	65	70	–	800-355-2583
41	37	32	28	23	18	73	76	77	296	73	78	75	83	80	91	73	87	$1.01	800-555-1514
52	53	53	33	29	26	70	69	77	142	61	60	69	71	70	85	58	63	–	800-663-8081
52	49	50	38	35	25	72	73	76	327	72	73	75	79	79	91	65	80	–	800-444-6222
69	65	61	45	39	35	75	76	81	293	71	71	76	82	78	90	63	71	–	973-244-8080
42	42	45	32	24	26	61	57	65	152	–	–	–	–	–	–	–	–	–	888-879-8471
–	–	–	–	–	–	–	–	–	–	71	74	75	77	75	90	69	72	–	888-476-8069

Accreditation status with NCQA (1/2002) is shown. Accreditation status with JCAHO (1/2002) is shown as follows: JCAHO=With commendation or with full standards compliance; JCAHO=With requirements for improvement. **Accreditation with the American**

Accreditation HealthCare Commission is shown as: AAHC. None=No accreditation action reported by any of the three accrediting organizations.

Plan Ratings

✓ means plan receives our top rating
Highest scores are in Blue
Lowest scores are in *Bold Italic*
"—" means no data

Footnotes are on page 56

	Doctors' overall rating of plan for patient care (% favorable)	Members' overall rating of plan (% favorable)	Key performance measures		Accreditation status**	% of members who had a problem (lower is better)	
			Direct measures of actual care for which plan was among the best or worst plans (see codes below)*				
			Best	Worst or not reported		"Big" problem getting referrals/tests/care	Called/wrote plan with complaint or problem
Average for all plans	57	60				9	20
New Mexico							
Blue Cross and Blue Shield of New Mexico (POS) (All or most of NM)	–	61	None	abfghik	None	*11*	*25*
Cimarron Health Plan (All or most of New Mexico)	–	*48*	c	abdhij	Accredited	*17*	20
HMO New Mexico[2] (HMO) (All or most of New Mexico)	–	*52*	dk	cegi	Commendable	11	24
Lovelace Health Systems (All or most of New Mexico)	–	61	cj	fk	Commendable[11]	9	20
Presbyterian Health Plan (All or most of New Mexico)	–	58	c	fghik	Commendable[12]	*12*	18
New York							
Aetna U.S. Healthcare (NYC, Long Island, Downstate NY, Bing., Syr.)	*43*	59	bh	df	Excellent	9	18
Atlantis Health Plan (NYC, Long Island, Westchester & Rockland cos)	56	–	–	–	None	–	–
✓ BlueCross Blue Shield of Western NY/Community Blue (Western NY)	61	68	cgh	None	Excellent	5	14
BlueShield of Northeastern New York (Northeastern New York)	–	57	fghi	None	Excellent	5	22
✓ Capital District Physicians' Health Plan (Eastern Upstate New York)	–	76	abehi	None	Excellent	3	16
CIGNA HealthCare of NY (NYC, Long Island, and Downstate NY)	*45*	*46*	c	dfi	Commendable	*12*	*29*
✓ Empire BlueCross BlueShield[15] (HMO) (Eastern and Downstate NY)	73	61	None	e	Excellent	9	22
✓ Excellus Health Plan/Blue Choice[2] (Rochester area)	79	72	acdefhik	None	Excellent	4	10
GHI HMO Select (HMO) (NYC and eastern New York)	58	*47*	–	–	None	9	*35*
Health Net of the Northeast[1] (NYC, Long Island, and Downstate NY)	60	63	–	–	None	5	22
Healthfirst New York (New York City)	47	–	–	–	None	–	–
HIP Health Plan (NYC, Long Island, and Downstate New York)	*39*	59	chik	ef	Commendable	11	14
HMO Blue[2] (HMO) (Rome, Utica, and Watertown areas)	–	59	defh	g	Excellent	7	*28*
✓ HMO-CNY[2] (HMO) (Central New York)	–	61	bdefhijk	None	Excellent	6	24
✓ Independent Health (HMO) (Western New York)	69	71	abceik	g	Excellent	5	11
MagnaHealth (NYC, Long Island, and Westchester County)	61	–	–	–	None	–	–
MDNY Healthcare (Long Island)	48	–	–	–	None	–	–
✓ MVP Health Care (HMO) (Central and eastern Upstate NY & So. Tier)	–	71	–	–	Commendable	4	15
✓ Oxford Health Plans (NYC, Long Island, and Downstate New York)	64	61	gj	None	Excellent	9	15
✓ Preferred Care (Rochester area)	58	75	defgij	None	Excellent	5	12
UnitedHealthcare of NY (NYC, Long Island, and Downstate NY)	66	*54*	c	dehik	Commendable	8	*28*
UnitedHealthcare of Upstate New York (Upstate New York)	–	64	dj	None	None	5	23
Univera Healthcare Central New York[2] (Syracuse area)	–	63	bcjk	None	Accredited	6	19
✓ Univera Healthcare Western New York[2] (Western New York)	57	67	abcdeghik	None	Excellent	5	14
Vytra Health Plans (Long Island and Queens)	52	66	fgk	None	None	7	21

*Assuring proper prevention and screening: a=Adolescent immunizations; b=Childhood immunizations; c=Chlamydia screening in sexually active women; d=Breast cancer screening; e=Cervical cancer screening. Assuring proper treatment: f=Beta blocker treatment after a heart attack; g=Cholesterol management (two measures); h=Controlling high blood pressure; i=Comprehensive diabetes care (six measures); j=Use of appropriate asthma medication; k=Followup after hospitalization for mental illness. "Best" or "worst" indicates plan's scores were in either the top or bottom 25 percent of benchmark plans.

Detailed performance measures

Ratings by doctors (% favorable)										Ratings by members (% favorable)									
Ability of patients to see appropriate specialists	Ability of patients to get needed tests and treatments	Ability of patients to get appropriate drugs	Plan's programs to help doctors give better care	How plan helps doctors follow up with patients	Incentives plan gives doctors affecting quality of care	Quality of primary care physicians affiliated with plan	Quality of specialists affiliated with plan	Quality of hospitals doctors can refer to within the plan	Number of doctors rating plan on the survey	Overall health care	Personal doctors	Specialist doctors	No problem getting referrals/tests/care	Getting care quickly	How well doctors communicate	Plan's customer service	Plan's claims processing	Estimated cost index for single person	Plan's phone number
56	56	52	42	36	30	72	76	78		73	75	77	79	78	90	67	81	$1.00	800-999-9999
–	–	–	–	–	–	–	–	–	–	74	75	80	75	74	92	65	86	–	800-835-8699
–	–	–	–	–	–	–	–	–	–	64	72	73	66	66	90	63	83	$0.91	505-342-4660
–	–	–	–	–	–	–	–	–	–	68	74	76	76	76	91	61	79	–	800-835-8699
–	–	–	–	–	–	–	–	–	–	71	75	72	80	77	89	66	80	$0.94	800-877-7526
–	–	–	–	–	–	–	–	–	–	64	66	74	74	68	85	67	83	$0.87	800-356-2219
43	46	44	38	28	24	66	68	76	390	70	74	75	80	75	89	71	75	$0.96[13]	800-323-9930
54	57	56	47	42	38	67	69	73	66	–	–	–	–	–	–	–	–	–	212-747-0877
64	59	50	54	45	31	86	92	85	87	73	74	80	88	84	93	73	92	–	800-544-2583
–	–	–	–	–	–	–	–	–	–	78	79	76	87	86	95	67	82	–	800-459-7587
–	–	–	–	–	–	–	–	–	–	76	78	81	87	84	92	74	91	$0.97[14]	888-258-0477
50	49	45	37	30	29	67	69	74	310	65	67	65	70	70	88	58	68	–	800-832-3211
71	69	64	54	47	43	82	84	84	363	75	76	75	81	80	90	66	81	–	212-476-1000
77	79	63	53	39	21	96	96	94	141	79	76	80	89	87	93	73	95	$1.07	800-847-1200
64	64	59	47	39	37	69	69	76	274	67	72	70	75	79	89	59	64	$1.06[16]	877-244-4466
62	58	56	40	35	31	75	73	77	545	74	76	77	83	78	91	67	76	$1.35	800-909-3447
46	48	50	36	33	31	64	64	68	150	–	–	–	–	–	–	–	–	–	888-260-1010
38	39	37	32	26	21	52	59	62	269	63	69	65	77	66	84	69	67	$0.91	800-447-8255
–	–	–	–	–	–	–	–	–	–	75	76	80	83	83	91	64	81	$1.02	800-722-7884
–	–	–	–	–	–	–	–	–	–	79	80	82	84	86	94	65	87	$1.08	800-462-6615
74	72	55	62	56	40	88	96	82	94	78	74	82	89	84	94	81	93	$0.80	716-631-3001
61	60	58	43	35	32	71	74	75	180	–	–	–	–	–	–	–	–	–	800-352-6465
48	46	47	40	31	30	68	67	71	128	–	–	–	–	–	–	–	–	–	631-454-1900
–	–	–	–	–	–	–	–	–	–	76	77	79	86	86	94	80	91	$0.97[17]	888-687-6277
63	60	55	50	40	36	79	81	82	443	75	78	74	82	76	89	70	82	–	800-444-6222
57	64	55	37	26	17	94	94	93	135	83	78	79	88	88	95	79	94	$0.99	800-800-7169
69	68	60	48	40	37	79	78	79	419	67	73	72	82	75	90	65	71	–	800-339-5380
–	–	–	–	–	–	–	–	–	–	79	80	83	90	84	93	62	78	–	800-339-5380
–	–	–	–	–	–	–	–	–	–	77	74	78	85	84	92	70	87	$1.06	888-747-6400
61	63	47	55	45	28	79	86	78	85	76	76	78	87	85	92	71	88	$0.85	800-427-8490
55	55	50	44	36	31	73	73	76	145	76	74	74	84	77	90	73	81	$1.13	800-406-0806

Accreditation status with NCQA (1/2002) is shown. Accreditation status with JCAHO (1/2002) is shown as follows: JCAHO=With commendation or with full standards compliance; JCAHO=With requirements for improvement. **Accreditation with the American **Accreditation HealthCare Commission is shown as: AAHC. None=No accreditation action** reported by any of the three accrediting organizations.

Plan Ratings

✓ means plan receives our top rating
Highest scores are in Blue
Lowest scores are in *Bold Italic*
"—" means no data

Footnotes are on page 56

	Doctors' overall rating of plan for patient care (% favorable)	Members' overall rating of plan (% favorable)	Key performance measures: Direct measures of actual care for which plan was among the best or worst plans (see codes below)* — Best	Worst or not reported	Accreditation status**	% of members who had a problem (lower is better): "Big" problem getting referrals/tests/care	Called/wrote plan with complaint or problem
Average for all plans	57	60				9	20
North Carolina							
Aetna U.S. Healthcare (Charlotte and Triangle areas)	*40*	*53*	None	None	None	*11*	*28*
✓ BlueCross BlueShield of NC/Personal Care (All or most of NC)	72	64	abdeh	k	Excellent	7	17
CIGNA HealthCare of North Carolina[18] (All of North Carolina)	*42*	61	bdef	hk	Commendable	10	*25*
Coventry Health Care Carolinas (Charlotte area)	*32*	*49*	None[19]	de[19]	None	10	*32*
Doctors Health Plan (Charlotte, Fayetteville, Triangle, Wilmington)	47	63	—	—	None	8	*26*
One Health Plan (HMO) (Charlotte, Greensboro, Triangle, Winst.-Sal.)	—	*48*	None[19]	e[19]	None	8	*31*
Optimum Choice of the Carolinas (Char., Greens., Tri., Winst.-Sal.)	*40*	55	None[19]	ad[19]	None	10	*37*
PARTNERS National Health Plan of NC[2] (All or most of NC)	55	62	deghi	j	Excellent	9	22
✓ UnitedHealthcare of North Carolina (Most of North Carolina)	73	74	de	hk	Excellent	5	20
WellPath Select[2] (Most of North Carolina)	*42*	64	be[19]	None[19]	None	7	18
Ohio							
Aetna U.S. Healthcare (Most of Ohio)	56	*54*	d	i	Commendable	7	*32*
✓ Anthem Blue Cross and Blue Shield (Most of Ohio)	63	63	None	e	Excellent	7	*26*
✓ AultCare (HMO) (Canton area)	—	84	—	—	None	2	20
CIGNA HealthCare Ohio (Most of Ohio)	56	55	None	None	Excellent	10	*30*
Family Health Plan (Northwestern Ohio)	—	62	chi	abdegjk	Commendable	7	*24*
✓ HAP (HMO) (Northwestern Ohio)	70	68	abcdfhjk	None	Excellent	8	13
✓ The Health Plan of the Upper Ohio Valley (HMO) (Southeastern Ohio)	—	77	de	bcfghij	Excellent	—	—
✓ HealthAmerica (HMO) (Eastern Ohio)	52	74	abdefghik	None	Excellent	6	17
HealthAmerica (POS) (Eastern Ohio)	52	60	abdfghik	None	Excellent	6	17
HMO Health Ohio (All of Ohio)	55	59	—	—	None	5	*29*
HomeTown Health Network (HMO) (Eastern Ohio)	—	68	None	cegj	None	7	*26*
Humana/ChoiceCare (Southern and central Ohio)	61	69	fj	None	Commendable	6	19
Kaiser Permanente Ohio (HMO) (Akron, Canton, and Cleveland areas)	53	62	bcdfik	j	Excellent	9	12
Nationwide Health Plans (All of Ohio)	70	—	—	—	None	—	—
One Health Plan of Ohio (Parts of Ohio)	61	—	—	—	None	—	—
✓ Paramount Health Care (HMO) (Northwestern Ohio)	—	73	e	ghj	Commendable	5	15
QualChoice (Northeastern Ohio)	79	—	—	—	Excellent	—	—
✓ SummaCare (Northeastern Ohio)	65	68	None	fgij	Excellent	8	22
SuperMed HMO (Northeastern Ohio)	76	59	—	—	Commendable	5	*29*
✓ UnitedHealthcare of Ohio (Central and southeastern Ohio)	62	61	defh	None	Excellent	5	20
UnitedHealthcare of Ohio (Northern Ohio)	76	55	None	eghij	Commendable	7	*28*
✓ UnitedHealthcare of Ohio (Southwestern Ohio)	61	62	ef	None	Excellent	5	23

***Assuring proper prevention and screening:** a=Adolescent immunizations; b=Childhood immunizations; c=Chlamydia screening in sexually active women; d=Breast cancer screening; e=Cervical cancer screening. **Assuring proper treatment:** f=Beta blocker treatment after a heart attack; g=Cholesterol management (two measures); h=Controlling high blood pressure; i=Comprehensive diabetes care (six measures); j=Use of appropriate asthma medication; k=Followup after hospitalization for mental illness. "Best" or "worst" indicates plan's scores were in either the top or bottom 25 percent of benchmark plans.

Detailed performance measures

Ratings by doctors (% favorable)										Ratings by members (% favorable)									
Ability of patients to see appropriate specialists	Ability of patients to get needed tests and treatments	Ability of patients to get appropriate drugs	Plan's programs to help doctors give better care	How plan helps doctors follow up with patients	Incentives plan gives doctors affecting quality of care	Quality of primary care physicians affiliated with plan	Quality of specialists affiliated with plan	Quality of hospitals doctors can refer to within the plan	Number of doctors rating plan on the survey	Overall health care	Personal doctors	Specialist doctors	No problem getting referrals/tests/care	Getting care quickly	How well doctors communicate	Plan's customer service	Plan's claims processing	Estimated cost index for single person	Plan's phone number
56	56	52	42	36	30	72	76	78		73	75	77	79	78	90	67	81	$1.00	800-999-9999
46	47	42	31	33	21	74	83	85	91	76	78	76	75	80	91	60	66	–	800-323-9930
70	69	66	40	37	33	85	86	90	155	74	78	80	84	81	91	71	86	–	800-250-3630
39	40	40	30	26	23	77	80	84	153	74	78	79	77	81	92	66	81	–	800-832-3211
31	37	40	26	24	27	70	66	70	34	76	77	79	74	81	91	58	67	–	800-889-1947
47	53	50	27	25	21	67	71	79	73	75	77	81	76	81	91	71	78	–	877-855-3034
–	–	–	–	–	–	–	–	–	–	68	72	80	75	79	89	56	60	–	800-663-8081
36	40	45	21	22	20	69	79	82	63	70	70	77	73	81	90	64	69	–	800-347-1965
47	57	47	37	34	31	76	81	80	145	76	78	81	80	82	92	68	82	–	800-942-5695
73	74	69	51	43	36	82	88	89	146	80	83	81	90	83	92	77	88	–	800-772-1180
47	48	50	30	28	26	64	72	81	109	81	82	82	79	83	93	70	82	–	800-935-7284
51	53	51	40	35	30	80	79	83	223	75	77	79	80	82	92	63	76	$1.13[6]	800-323-9930
66	63	62	51	40	35	83	83	86	194	75	74	81	83	83	92	65	84	$1.06	800-438-9672
–	–	–	–	–	–	–	–	–	–	83	80	86	91	89	93	84	95	$0.79	800-344-8858
54	53	52	40	33	30	81	83	83	171	73	72	76	76	80	91	64	80	–	800-832-3211
–	–	–	–	–	–	–	–	–	–	74	72	77	82	80	90	68	85	–	800-231-8274
60	62	60	61	52	43	81	89	86	177	71	74	76	82	77	89	72	82	$0.99	800-422-4641
–	–	–	–	–	–	–	–	–	–	84	80	88	–	85	94	82	96	$0.98	800-624-6961
52	46	33	32	26	19	80	81	77	68	82	78	79	86	85	93	72	87	$0.94	800-788-8445
52	46	33	32	26	19	80	81	77	68	82	77	82	86	84	93	67	79	–	800-788-8445
46	48	51	27	24	24	65	70	74	85	75	73	79	79	81	92	60	79	$1.06	800-245-5272
–	–	–	–	–	–	–	–	–	–	80	76	83	83	86	92	70	85	–	800-426-9013
53	57	53	33	38	22	78	79	82	87	70	68	75	85	79	90	75	88	–	800-448-6262
37	53	55	48	48	40	53	55	69	34	69	73	73	83	80	88	76	74	$0.96	800-686-7100
68	62	60	41	38	37	80	82	84	106	–	–	–	–	–	–	–	–	–	800-940-3553
56	57	52	36	28	28	72	75	75	69	–	–	–	–	–	–	–	–	–	800-663-8081
–	–	–	–	–	–	–	–	–	–	80	76	82	88	84	95	73	91	$1.07	800-462-3589
74	74	64	64	51	48	89	90	82	81	–	–	–	–	–	–	–	–	–	800-260-2643
63	59	58	59	44	44	74	78	75	37	78	80	80	81	83	93	68	86	$0.83	800-996-8701
63	67	60	48	38	36	84	83	83	67	75	73	79	79	81	92	60	79	$1.17	800-245-5272
71	67	62	56	52	36	85	86	85	55	76	75	78	87	84	91	69	86	–	800-328-8835
75	75	67	59	51	44	89	90	91	74	75	77	78	85	82	91	64	75	–	800-468-5001
63	59	64	38	29	24	80	76	76	59	77	78	77	88	82	91	68	81	$1.21	800-231-2198

Accreditation status with NCQA (1/2002) is shown. Accreditation status with JCAHO (1/2002) is shown as follows: JCAHO=With commendation or with full standards compliance; JCAHO=With requirements for improvement. **Accreditation with the American Accreditation HealthCare Commission is shown as: AAHC. None=No accreditation action reported by any of the three accrediting organizations.

Plan Ratings

✓ means plan receives our top rating
Highest scores are in **Blue**
Lowest scores are in ***Bold Italic***
"—" means no data

Footnotes are on page 56

	Key performance measures						
	Doctors' overall rating of plan for patient care (% favorable)	Members' overall rating of plan (% favorable)	Direct measures of actual care for which plan was among the best or worst plans (see codes below)*		Accreditation status**	% of members who had a problem (lower is better)	
			Best	Worst or not reported		"Big" problem getting referrals/tests/care	Called/wrote plan with complaint or problem
Average for all plans	57	60				9	20
Oklahoma							
PacifiCare of Oklahoma (HMO) (Oklahoma City and Tulsa areas)	–	60	None	cfgh	Excellent	*15*	19
Oregon							
Health Net Health Plan of Oregon[20] (Most of western Oregon)	47	–	–	–	None	–	–
✓ Kaiser Permanente Northwest (HMO) (Corvallis, Portland, Salem)	78	62	abcfgik	None	Excellent	*11*	11
PacifiCare of Oregon (HMO) (Corvallis, Portland, and Salem areas)	47	*54*	i	ch	Excellent	*13*	18
✓ Providence Health Plans (Corvallis, Eugene, Portland, Salem areas)	73	60	di	h	Excellent	10	17
Regence HMO Oregon (Eastern Oregon)	79	*50*	k	abcghij	Commendable	–	–
Pennsylvania							
✓ Aetna U.S. Healthcare (HMO) (Southeastern Pennsylvania)	57	63	abij	h	Excellent	6	15
Aetna U.S. Healthcare (POS) (Southeastern Pennsylvania)	57	*54*	abij	ch	Excellent	8	15
Aetna U.S. Healthcare (HMO) (Western Pennsylvania)	*35*	59	abfi	cdh	Excellent	7	19
Aetna U.S. Healthcare (POS) (Western Pennsylvania)	*35*	55	ab	cdgh	Excellent	8	17
AmeriHealth HMO of New Jersey (Southeastern Pennsylvania)	*43*	58	bf	j	Excellent	7	*26*
CIGNA HealthCare of Pennsylvania (Southeastern Pennsylvania)	52	*49*	abfg	None	Excellent	10	*27*
Coventry Health Care (Southeastern Pennsylvania)	*36*	63	acd	gjk	None	6	*28*
✓ First Priority Health (Northeastern Pennsylvania)	–	62	aghj	cd	Excellent	6	17
✓ Geisinger Health Plan (Central and northeastern Pennsylvania)	–	*71*	abfghi	None	Excellent	7	*12*
Health Net of the Northeast[20] (SE PA, Scranton/Wilkes-Barre area)	*42*	58	–	–	None	6	23
✓ HealthAmerica (HMO) (Central and western Pennsylvania)	52	*74*	abdefghik	None	Excellent	6	17
HealthAmerica (POS) (Central and western Pennsylvania)	52	60	abdfghik	None	Excellent	6	17
✓ HealthGuard (Harrisburg, Lancaster, Reading, and York areas)	–	*71*	gi	bfk	Excellent	6	15
✓ Keystone Health Plan Central (HMO) (Central Pennsylvania)	–	*74*	adghi	c	Excellent	7	14
Keystone Health Plan East (Eastern Pennsylvania)	*40*	65	abi	cde	Excellent	8	13
✓ Keystone Health Plan West (Western Pennsylvania)	79	69	afghi	None	Excellent	6	14
✓ NewAlliance Health Plan (Northwestern Pennsylvania)	–	60	aej	ck	Excellent	6	13
✓ UPMC Health Plan (Western Pennsylvania)	87	63	ade	j	None	7	*24*
Puerto Rico							
✓ Triple-S (HMO) (All of Puerto Rico)	–	84	–	–	None	3	10
Rhode Island							
Aetna U.S. Healthcare (All or most of Rhode Island)	*44*	*52*	abh	None	Commendable	9	*24*
✓ BlueCHiP (All of Rhode Island)	57	67	eh	fij	Excellent	6	17
✓ BlueCross BlueShield of MA/HMO Blue (All or most of RI)	84	*74*	abdefk	None	Excellent	4	15

*Assuring proper prevention and screening:** a=Adolescent immunizations; b=Childhood immunizations; c=Chlamydia screening in sexually active women; d=Breast cancer screening; e=Cervical cancer screening. **Assuring proper treatment:** f=Beta blocker treatment after a heart attack; g=Cholesterol management (two measures); h=Controlling high blood pressure; i=Comprehensive diabetes care (six measures); j=Use of appropriate asthma medication; k=Followup after hospitalization for mental illness. "Best" or "worst" indicates plan's scores were in either the top or bottom 25 percent of benchmark plans.

Detailed performance measures

Ability of patients to see appropriate specialists	Ability of patients to get needed tests and treatments	Ability of patients to get appropriate drugs	Plan's programs to help doctors give better care	How plan helps doctors follow up with patients	Incentives plan gives doctors affecting quality of care	Quality of primary care physicians affiliated with plan	Quality of specialists affiliated with plan	Quality of hospitals doctors can refer to within the plan	Number of doctors rating plan on the survey	Overall health care	Personal doctors	Specialist doctors	No problem getting referrals/tests/care	Getting care quickly	How well doctors communicate	Plan's customer service	Plan's claims processing	Estimated cost index for single person	Plan's phone number
56	56	52	42	36	30	72	76	78		73	75	77	79	78	90	67	81	$1.00	800-999-9999
–	–	–	–	–	–	–	–	–		71	70	74	71	76	88	67	86	$0.83	800-825-9355
54	55	50	33	26	18	80	81	88	85	–	–	–	–	–	–	–	–	–	503-802-7000
71	74	85	81	71	66	85	83	76	55	69	76	72	81	77	89	77	84	$1.05	800-813-2000
39	43	48	34	26	22	73	82	89	106	66	68	76	72	76	89	63	89	$1.29	800-932-3004
66	72	71	56	52	35	92	94	90	110	68	69	76	77	79	86	68	88	–	800-878-4445
77	78	73	57	48	39	92	93	92	114	71	72	79	–	82	92	60	85	–	800-228-0978
57	51	43	39	31	24	84	90	88	217	77	80	79	85	82	92	71	85	–	800-323-9930
57	51	43	39	31	24	84	90	88	217	72	77	74	82	81	92	64	83	–	800-323-9930
33	30	39	31	19	16	68	73	66	81	75	81	78	81	84	92	68	84	–	800-323-9930
33	30	39	31	19	16	68	73	66	81	71	75	75	79	82	90	65	80	–	800-323-9930
43	42	40	30	27	21	64	64	70	403	73	76	77	83	82	91	67	77	$1.08	856-778-6500
53	51	45	30	30	26	80	83	86	133	73	73	76	78	82	92	60	75	–	800-832-3211
42	37	40	30	14	18	66	69	70	47	75	72	78	87	82	90	65	77	–	800-833-7423
–	–	–	–	–	–	–	–	–		75	78	79	85	86	94	71	89	–	800-822-8753
–	–	–	–	–	–	–	–	–		77	79	79	86	84	92	77	88	–	800-631-1656
39	32	28	20	17	16	65	66	72	96	76	80	81	80	83	93	64	82	$1.19	800-909-3447
52	46	33	32	26	19	80	81	77	68	82	78	79	86	85	93	72	87	$0.94	800-788-8445
52	46	33	32	26	19	80	81	77	68	82	77	82	86	84	93	67	79	–	800-788-8445
–	–	–	–	–	–	–	–	–		77	79	77	86	85	92	75	93	$0.87	800-822-0350
–	–	–	–	–	–	–	–	–		78	77	81	84	86	93	73	92	$1.16	800-622-2843
41	37	32	28	23	18	73	76	77	296	73	78	75	83	80	91	73	87	$1.01	800-555-1514
72	71	51	50	36	29	91	93	91	86	78	75	83	85	81	92	73	91	$1.15	800-544-6679
–	–	–	–	–	–	–	–	–		77	74	83	85	85	92	71	85	–	800-752-4165
89	84	61	68	58	46	92	95	93	108	76	77	81	87	80	93	66	82	–	888-876-2756
–	–	–	–	–	–	–	–	–		86	92	91	92	73	93	82	84	$0.73	877-357-9777
43	50	45	33	28	25	67	71	75	248	74	76	80	79	80	91	60	70	–	800-323-9930
59	62	47	37	29	24	83	88	86	150	81	80	82	85	84	93	71	84	$1.07	401-274-3500
79	83	70	62	53	53	89	93	94	247	76	74	79	89	83	92	76	90	–	800-262-2583

Accreditation status with NCQA (1/2002) is shown. Accreditation status with JCAHO (1/2002) is shown as follows: JCAHO=With commendation or with full standards compliance; JCAHO=With requirements for improvement. **Accreditation with the American **Accreditation HealthCare Commission is shown as: AAHC. None=No accreditation action** reported by any of the three accrediting organizations.

Plan Ratings

✓ means plan receives our top rating
Highest scores are in Blue
Lowest scores are in *Bold Italic*
"—" means no data

Footnotes are on page 56

	Doctors' overall rating of plan for patient care (% favorable)	Members' overall rating of plan (% favorable)	Direct measures of actual care for which plan was among the best or worst plans (see codes below)*		Accreditation status**	"Big" problem getting referrals/tests/care	Called/wrote plan with complaint or problem
			Best	Worst or not reported		(lower is better)	(lower is better)
Average for all plans	57	60				9	20
Rhode Island *(continued)*							
HMO New England (All or most of Rhode Island)	50	—	—	—	None	—	—
✓ Tufts Health Plan (HMO) (All or most of Rhode Island)	72	65	abcdefk	ghi	Excellent	8	15
✓ Tufts Health Plan (POS) (All or most of Rhode Island)	72	67	abcdfjk	ghi	Excellent	6	16
✓ UnitedHealthcare of New England (All of Rhode Island)	57	71	abck	None	Excellent	5	18
South Carolina							
Aetna U.S. Healthcare (B'fort, Charleston, Clmbia, Rock Hill, Spart.)	*40*	*53*	None	None	None	*11*	*28*
✓ Carolina Care Plan[21] (All or most of South Carolina)	—	66	af	ghik	Commendable	7	15
CIGNA HealthCare of South Carolina (All of South Carolina)	—	65	None	ghij	Excellent	10	19
✓ Companion HealthCare (All or most of South Carolina)		65	abdefi	chj	Excellent	7	19
Coventry Health Care Carolinas (Union and York counties)	*32*	*49*	None	de	None	10	*32*
Doctors Health Plan (York County)	47	63	—	—	None	8	*26*
One Health Plan (HMO) (York County)	—	*48*	None	e	None	8	*31*
PARTNERS Nat'l HP of NC[2] (Columbia, Grnville, Rock Hill, Spartan.)	55	62	deghi	j	Excellent	9	22
WellPath Select[2] (Anderson, Greenville, Rock Hill, Spartanburg)	*42*	64	be	None	None	7	18
South Dakota							
Exclusive Healthcare (Union County)	—	—	bek	None	Excellent	—	—
Sioux Valley Health Plan (HMO) (Most of South Dakota)	—	*48*	k	abj	JCAHO	6	22
Tennessee							
Aetna U.S. Healthcare (Central Tennessee)	*38*	*44*	eh	ac	Excellent	9	*30*
Aetna U.S. Healthcare (Memphis area)	—	59	None	abcdefghijk	Accredited	—	—
CIGNA HealthCare of Tennessee (Most of Tennessee)	*32*	59	None	ai	Commendable	*11*	23
HealthSpring[7] (Nashville area)	62	—	—	—	None	—	—
HMO Blue (All or most of Tennessee)	56	64	None	abcghij	Commendable	—	—
✓ John Deere Health Plan (HMO) (Eastern Tennessee)	—	72	defghijk	None	Excellent	5	14
One Health Plan of Tennessee (Memphis and Nashville areas)	55	—	—	—	None	—	—
✓ UnitedHealthcare of Tennessee (Most of Tennessee)	71	67	None	aghi	JCAHO	5	*27*
Texas							
Aetna U.S. Healthcare (Austin, Corpus Ch., El Paso, Hou., San Ant.)	53	*53*	None	a	Excellent	10	22
Aetna U.S. Healthcare (Dallas-Ft. Worth area)	52	*53*	None	af	Excellent	*12*	*26*
AmCare Health Plans (Most of Texas)	52	*47*	None[22]	bdehij[22]	None	10	25
Amil International (HMO) (Austin area)	—	59	None[22]	bcdehi[22]	None	*12*	22
CIGNA HealthCare of North Texas (Northern Texas)	*46*	57	bc[22]	None[22]	Commendable	9	21

*Assuring proper prevention and screening: a=Adolescent immunizations; b=Childhood immunizations; c=Chlamydia screening in sexually active women; d=Breast cancer screening; e=Cervical cancer screening. Assuring proper treatment: f=Beta blocker treatment after a heart attack; g=Cholesterol management (two measures); h=Controlling high blood pressure; i=Comprehensive diabetes care (six measures); j=Use of appropriate asthma medication; k=Followup after hospitalization for mental illness. "Best" or "worst" indicates plan's scores were in either the top or bottom 25 percent of benchmark plans.

Detailed performance measures																			
Ratings by doctors (% favorable)										Ratings by members (% favorable)									
Ability of patients to see appropriate specialists	Ability of patients to get needed tests and treatments	Ability of patients to get appropriate drugs	Plan's programs to help doctors give better care	How plan helps doctors follow up with patients	Incentives plan gives doctors affecting quality of care	Quality of primary care physicians affiliated with plan	Quality of specialists affiliated with plan	Quality of hospitals doctors can refer to within the plan	Number of doctors rating plan on the survey	Overall health care	Personal doctors	Specialist doctors	No problem getting referrals/tests/care	Getting care quickly	How well doctors communicate	Plan's customer service	Plan's claims processing	Estimated cost index for single person	Plan's phone number
56	56	52	42	36	30	72	76	78		73	75	77	79	78	90	67	81	$1.00	800-999-9999
51	61	52	40	26	21	80	81	79	30	–	–	–	–	–	–	–	–	–	800-331-0150
70	75	62	57	48	44	86	87	90	335	78	73	81	83	81	92	75	85	–	800-462-0224
70	75	62	57	48	44	86	87	90	335	78	78	83	86	84	94	73	82	–	800-843-1008
60	65	49	44	35	27	80	82	84	261	80	80	80	89	84	92	73	89	–	800-447-1245
46	47	42	31	33	21	74	83	85	91	76	78	76	75	80	91	60	66	–	800-323-9930
–	–	–	–	–	–	–	–	–	–	78	83	79	87	82	93	71	86	–	800-747-9995
–	–	–	–	–	–	–	–	–	–	76	82	81	80	79	93	72	82	–	800-832-3211
–	–	–	–	–	–	–	–	–	–	75	79	81	82	81	90	72	84	–	800-868-2528
31	37	40	26	24	27	70	66	70	34	76	77	79	74	81	91	58	67	–	800-889-1947
47	53	50	27	25	21	67	71	79	73	75	77	81	76	81	91	71	78	–	877-855-3034
–	–	–	–	–	–	–	–	–	–	68	72	80	75	79	89	56	60	–	800-663-8081
47	57	47	37	34	31	76	81	80	145	76	78	81	80	82	92	68	82	–	800-942-5695
47	48	50	30	28	26	64	72	81	109	81	82	82	79	83	93	70	82	–	800-935-7284
–	–	–	–	–	–	–	–	–	–	–	–	–	–	–	–	–	–	–	800-631-4333
–	–	–	–	–	–	–	–	–	–	76	78	82	88	84	93	62	82	–	605-333-1000
32	40	36	25	20	11	73	69	73	64	67	72	76	79	77	88	62	74	$1.06	800-323-9930
–	–	–	–	–	–	–	–	–	–	68	79	75	–	67	86	69	81	$0.90	800-323-9930
33	37	31	32	22	14	74	70	74	62	68	71	76	75	72	88	68	83	–	800-832-3211
54	59	54	40	38	26	89	83	87	52	–	–	–	–	–	–	–	–	–	800-881-9466
63	60	62	39	38	23	75	81	82	48	75	75	79	–	75	90	70	85	–	800-565-9140
–	–	–	–	–	–	–	–	–	–	81	79	81	89	86	93	72	92	–	800-224-6599
58	59	59	39	40	21	80	81	82	33	–	–	–	–	–	–	–	–	–	800-663-8081
76	74	74	46	45	35	91	90	92	58	80	80	81	88	79	92	66	81	–	800-695-1273
54	50	47	36	32	20	75	81	81	219	68	73	78	76	73	89	63	77	–	800-323-9930
50	54	55	41	38	29	74	73	78	131	72	74	79	73	75	89	62	73	–	800-323-9930
48	51	46	31	27	24	63	71	74	103	66	73	81	74	73	90	61	67	–	800-782-8373
–	–	–	–	–	–	–	–	–	–	72	72	81	66	77	90	67	79	–	888-349-2645
47	51	41	38	33	29	69	70	71	110	65	68	72	73	74	87	63	80	–	800-832-3211

Accreditation status with NCQA (1/2002) is shown. Accreditation status with JCAHO (1/2002) is shown as follows: JCAHO=With commendation or with full standards compliance; JCAHO=With requirements for improvement. **Accreditation with the American

Accreditation HealthCare Commission is shown as: AAHC. None=No accreditation action reported by any of the three accrediting organizations.

Plan Ratings

✓ means plan receives our top rating
Highest scores are in Blue
Lowest scores are in *Bold Italic*
"–" means no data

Footnotes are on page 56

	Doctors' overall rating of plan for patient care (% favorable)	Members' overall rating of plan (% favorable)	Key performance measures		Accreditation status**	% of members who had a problem (lower is better)	
			Direct measures of actual care for which plan was among the best or worst plans (see codes below)*				
			Best	Worst or not reported		"Big" problem getting referrals/tests/care	Called/wrote plan with complaint or problem
Average for all plans	57	60				9	20
Texas (continued)							
CIGNA HealthCare of South Texas (Southern Texas)	65	56	ch[22]	None[22]	Commendable	8	*24*
Community First Health Plans (HMO) (San Antonio area)	51	63	j	ck	None	*15*	19
FIRSTCARE (HMO) (Abilene area)	–	65	None	abdj	None	7	*10*
FIRSTCARE (HMO) (Amarillo area)	–	63	h	abegjk	None	8	*14*
FIRSTCARE (HMO) (Lubbock area)	–	64	None	abegj	None	7	*15*
FIRSTCARE (HMO) (Waco area)	–	*53*	g	abcdij	None	*11*	18
Heritage Health Plan (Northeastern Texas)	–	*71*	None	bi	None	8	17
HMO Blue, Central/South TX (HMO) (Most of southern and central TX)	54	56	cj[22]	None[22]	None	7	*24*
HMO Blue, El Paso (HMO) (El Paso area)	–	58	j[22]	dei[22]	None	9	23
HMO Blue, Northeast Texas (HMO) (Dallas-Ft. Worth area)	51	58	j[22]	bdeik[22]	None	9	23
HMO Blue, Southeast Texas (HMO) (Houston area)	64	59	cj[22]	bdehik[22]	None	10	*26*
HMO Blue, Southwest Texas (HMO) (Abilene and San Angelo areas)	–	60	j[22]	hik[22]	None	5	18
HMO Blue, Southwest Texas (HMO) (Midland area)	–	*51*	j[22]	dhi[22]	None	*11*	19
HMO Blue Texas (Austin area)	*38*	*53*	b[22]	cdik[22]	None	*11*	19
HMO Blue Texas (Beaumont and Lufkin areas)	–	59	None[22]	bcdeij[22]	None	7	*25*
HMO Blue Texas (Corpus Christi area)	–	*53*	h[22]	cdei[22]	None	9	*24*
HMO Blue Texas (Dallas-Ft. Worth area)	–	57	None[22]	bchik[22]	None	10	20
HMO Blue Texas (Houston area)	58	*52*	None[22]	bdei[22]	None	9	20
HMO Blue Texas (San Antonio area)	63	*50*	None[22]	bcdei[22]	None	*12*	*33*
HMO Blue, West Texas (HMO) (Texas Panhandle)	–	57	hj[22]	beik[22]	None	7	17
Humana Health Plan of Texas (HMO) (Austin area)	65	55	None	fg	None	*13*	23
Humana Health Plan of Texas (HMO) (Corpus Christi area)	–	61	None	bcegj	None	10	18
Humana Health Plan of Texas (HMO) (Houston area)	54	*48*	None	abdehij	None	*16*	*36*
Humana Health Plan of Texas (HMO) (San Antonio area)	*34*	*52*	h	cdj	None	*20*	*25*
Mercy Health Plans (HMO) (Laredo area)	–	75	None[22]	bdehij[22]	None	5	9
MethodistCare (HMO) (Southeastern Texas)	66	*53*	e[22]	bdij[22]	None	*11*	23
MetroWest Health Plan (Dallas-Ft. Worth area)	*43*	–	–	–	JCAHO	–	–
One Health Plan of Texas (HMO) (Central and southern Texas)	56	*53*	c[22]	bdehi[22]	None	*12*	21
One Health Plan of Texas (HMO) (Dallas-Ft. Worth area)	62	*53*	None[22]	dehi[22]	None	*11*	22
One Health Plan of Texas (HMO) (Houston area)	67	55	c[22]	bdehi[22]	None	*11*	23
PacifiCare of Texas (HMO) (Dallas-Ft. Worth area)	*21*	*44*	k	aceghi	Commendable	*20*	*27*
PacifiCare of Texas (HMO) (Houston area)	*35*	*46*	None	abcdehi	Commendable	*21*	*38*
PacifiCare of Texas (HMO) (San Antonio area)	*32*	64	k	cdegh	Commendable	*16*	21

*Assuring proper prevention and screening: a=Adolescent immunizations; b=Childhood immunizations; c=Chlamydia screening in sexually active women; d=Breast cancer screening; e=Cervical cancer screening. Assuring proper treatment: f=Beta blocker treatment after a heart attack; g=Cholesterol management (two measures); h=Controlling high blood pressure; i=Comprehensive diabetes care (six measures); j=Use of appropriate asthma medication; k=Followup after hospitalization for mental illness. "Best" or "worst" indicates plan's scores were in either the top or bottom 25 percent of benchmark plans.

Detailed performance measures

Ratings by doctors (% favorable)										Ratings by members (% favorable)									
Ability of patients to see appropriate specialists	Ability of patients to get needed tests and treatments	Ability of patients to get appropriate drugs	Plan's programs to help doctors give better care	How plan helps doctors follow up with patients	Incentives plan gives doctors affecting quality of care	Quality of primary care physicians affiliated with plan	Quality of specialists affiliated with plan	Quality of hospitals doctors can refer to within the plan	Number of doctors rating plan on the survey	Overall health care	Personal doctors	Specialist doctors	No problem getting referrals/tests/care	Getting care quickly	How well doctors communicate	Plan's customer service	Plan's claims processing	Estimated cost index for single person	Plan's phone number
56	56	52	42	36	30	72	76	78		73	75	77	79	78	90	67	81	$1.00	800-999-9999
52	55	50	44	35	28	71	80	83	94	65	72	73	74	72	88	65	80	—	800-832-3211
49	52	46	34	35	25	61	71	72	61	71	79	75	68	67	89	72	68	—	210-358-6070
—	—	—	—	—	—	—	—	—	—	79	78	80	84	84	94	75	94	$1.23	800-884-4901
—	—	—	—	—	—	—	—	—	—	76	78	81	82	81	94	73	91	$1.23	800-884-4901
—	—	—	—	—	—	—	—	—	—	78	81	84	79	81	93	74	89	$1.23	800-884-4901
—	—	—	—	—	—	—	—	—	—	78	81	82	76	79	93	67	80	$1.12	800-884-4901
—	—	—	—	—	—	—	—	—	—	84	84	72	83	83	93	70	87	—	903-531-4447
53	60	51	37	37	29	64	66	83	68	70	75	77	75	74	88	64	79	—	877-299-2377
—	—	—	—	—	—	—	—	—	—	66	70	71	70	63	85	64	75	—	877-299-2377
52	50	50	41	34	34	70	71	78	96	69	67	79	73	73	86	64	74	—	877-299-2377
53	51	54	30	32	26	77	80	83	55	70	71	71	73	72	86	62	71	—	877-299-2377
—	—	—	—	—	—	—	—	—	—	74	74	82	82	76	91	66	82	—	877-299-2377
—	—	—	—	—	—	—	—	—	—	70	73	72	75	77	88	61	79	—	877-299-2377
47	56	46	30	29	24	62	56	81	34	65	70	74	71	73	87	64	75	—	877-299-2377
—	—	—	—	—	—	—	—	—	—	70	77	77	75	77	89	68	78	—	877-299-2377
—	—	—	—	—	—	—	—	—	—	70	71	78	72	75	90	61	78	—	877-299-2377
—	—	—	—	—	—	—	—	—	—	66	73	76	74	72	87	67	77	—	877-299-2377
54	54	58	36	33	32	70	72	81	93	67	72	70	73	71	88	66	74	—	877-299-2377
58	62	57	43	40	29	69	77	86	57	66	74	70	66	69	86	62	63	—	877-299-2377
—	—	—	—	—	—	—	—	—	—	73	77	78	78	76	92	67	81	—	877-299-2377
69	69	40	39	36	23	74	72	74	31	64	73	74	73	76	89	60	75	—	800-448-6262
—	—	—	—	—	—	—	—	—	—	71	69	79	77	76	87	71	85	—	800-448-6262
45	47	44	35	30	24	72	77	79	78	59	66	67	67	70	83	59	68	—	800-448-6262
33	31	26	31	28	21	40	56	67	71	61	71	74	62	69	84	69	75	$0.82	800-448-6262
—	—	—	—	—	—	—	—	—	—	81	84	81	81	75	94	77	87	—	800-617-3433
61	64	58	47	33	37	77	84	84	79	61	69	73	69	68	87	65	66	—	888-955-4200
29	39	35	32	35	29	57	57	61	28	—	—	—	—	—	—	—	—	—	817-665-5100
46	52	43	49	42	35	58	67	84	48	66	67	71	67	74	86	62	75	—	800-663-8081
69	72	64	41	40	41	82	78	83	60	67	67	71	69	73	84	59	73	—	800-663-8081
57	64	65	34	36	36	75	87	89	51	63	75	66	75	70	86	63	73	—	800-663-8081
20	22	18	16	14	13	50	45	51	112	70	73	80	61	71	89	53	68	$0.81	800-825-9355
32	37	23	23	16	17	66	56	68	65	63	69	67	60	67	85	60	60	$0.81	800-825-9355
33	34	25	27	26	12	44	59	58	75	73	77	76	70	76	88	70	75	$0.81	800-825-9355

Accreditation status with NCQA (1/2002) is shown. Accreditation status with JCAHO (1/2002) is shown as follows: JCAHO=With commendation or with full standards compliance; JCAHO=With requirements for improvement. **Accreditation with the American

Accreditation HealthCare Commission is shown as: AAHC. None=No accreditation action reported by any of the three accrediting organizations.

Plan Ratings

✓ means plan receives our top rating
Highest scores are in Blue
Lowest scores are in *Bold Italic*
"—" means no data

Footnotes are on page 56

Key performance measures

Plan	Doctors' overall rating of plan for patient care (% favorable)	Members' overall rating of plan (% favorable)	Direct measures of actual care for which plan was among the best or worst plans (see codes below)* — Best	Worst or not reported	Accreditation status**	"Big" problem getting referrals/tests/care	Called/wrote plan with complaint or problem
Average for all plans	57	60				9	20
Texas (continued)							
Parkland Community Health Plan (HMO) (Dallas area)	—	67	None	abdefj	None	9	9
✓ Scott & White Health Plan (HMO) (Austin and Waco areas)	—	81	defghi	cj	Excellent	7	9
Seton Health Plan (Austin and Waco areas)	71	—	—	—	JCAHO	—	—
✓ UnitedHealthcare of Texas (Austin, San Antonio, and Waco areas)	74	64	e	adgjk	Excellent	9	19
UnitedHealthcare of Texas (Dallas-Ft. Worth area)	76	60	None	abdfghi	Commendable	8	18
UnitedHealthcare of Texas (Southeastern and southern Texas)	82	64	None	abfghi	Commendable	6	*25*
Valley Baptist Health Plan (HMO) (Harlingen area)	—	69	ch[22]	bj[22]	None	7	10
Utah							
Altius Health Plans (Wasatch Front area)	64	*49*	—	—	None	10	*30*
CIGNA HealthCare (Wasatch Front area)	57	*46*	—	—	None	—	—
Intermountain Health Care (Most of Utah)	93	61	—	—	Commendable	—	—
Regence BlueCross BlueShield of UT/HealthWise (All or most of UT)	87	*51*	—	—	None	—	—
SelectMed (Most of Utah)	79	—	—	—	Commendable	—	—
UnitedHealthcare of Utah (Northern Utah)	71	*51*	—	—	JCAHO	—	—
University of Utah Health Network (Wasatch Front area)	—	58	—	—	None	—	—
Vermont							
BlueCross BlueShield of Vermont (POS) (All of Vermont)	—	*54*	acdeij	bf	None	7	*34*
✓ Harvard Pilgrim Health Care of New England (So. and eastern VT)	—	65	bdjk	None	Commendable	7	18
HMO New England (All or most of Vermont)	50	—	—	—	None	—	—
✓ MVP Health Care (HMO) (All of Vermont)	—	64	ghi	c	Commendable	4	17
The Vermont Health Plan (All of Vermont)	—	*52*	cdeijk	f	None	8	*27*
Virginia							
Aetna U.S. Healthcare (Northern Virginia)	*39*	*48*	bfh	cg	Commendable	*12*	23
Capital Care/CareFirst (Northern Virginia)	63	58	bdj	h	Excellent	9	23
CIGNA HealthCare Mid-Atlantic (Northern Virginia)	50	*48*	bch	i	Excellent	*13*	22
CIGNA HealthCare of Virginia (Most of Virginia)	—	56	beh	None	Commendable	9	21
HealthKeepers (Most of Virginia)	*44*	58	beh	None	Excellent	8	*16*
✓ John Deere Health Plan (HMO) (Southwestern Virginia)	—	72	defghijk	None	Excellent	5	14
Kaiser Foundation HP Mid-Atlantic States (HMO) (Northern VA)	56	60	abcef	None	Commendable	10	*13*
M.D. IPA (Most of Virginia)	50	70	bhj	f	Excellent	7	20
✓ Optima Health Plan (HMO) (Southeastern Virginia)	84	70	None	bcghij	Excellent	—	—
✓ Optima Health Plan (POS) (Southeastern Virginia)	84	68	e	bcghij	Excellent	—	—

*Assuring proper prevention and screening: a=Adolescent immunizations; b=Childhood immunizations; c=Chlamydia screening in sexually active women; d=Breast cancer screening; e=Cervical cancer screening. Assuring proper treatment: f=Beta blocker treatment after a heart attack; g=Cholesterol management (two measures); h=Controlling high blood pressure; i=Comprehensive diabetes care (six measures); j=Use of appropriate asthma medication; k=Followup after hospitalization for mental illness. "Best" or "worst" indicates plan's scores were in either the top or bottom 25 percent of benchmark plans.

Detailed performance measures

Ratings by doctors (% favorable)										Ratings by members (% favorable)									
Ability of patients to see appropriate specialists	Ability of patients to get needed tests and treatments	Ability of patients to get appropriate drugs	Plan's programs to help doctors give better care	How plan helps doctors follow up with patients	Incentives plan gives doctors affecting quality of care	Quality of primary care physicians affiliated with plan	Quality of specialists affiliated with plan	Quality of hospitals doctors can refer to within the plan	Number of doctors rating plan on the survey	Overall health care	Personal doctors	Specialist doctors	No problem getting referrals/tests/care	Getting care quickly	How well doctors communicate	Plan's customer service	Plan's claims processing	Estimated cost index for single person	Plan's phone number
56	56	52	42	36	30	72	76	78		73	75	77	79	78	90	67	81	$1.00	800-999-9999
–	–	–	–	–	–	–	–	–	–	76	77	83	79	71	90	64	81	–	888-672-2277
–	–	–	–	–	–	–	–	–	–	82	84	82	87	82	93	79	96	–	800-321-7947
81	77	63	40	50	39	76	81	77	31	–	–	–	–	–	–	–	–	–	800-749-7404
78	72	62	54	49	41	76	83	84	93	69	75	76	83	78	90	66	84	–	800-411-1145
77	77	70	61	58	51	83	83	86	112	70	74	78	83	76	88	66	80	–	800-842-2481
79	79	79	56	48	42	87	92	92	100	71	75	78	86	75	89	63	81	–	713-961-4300
–	–	–	–	–	–	–	–	–	–	74	80	73	76	76	91	78	85	–	956-389-2273
67	65	57	38	30	25	82	92	88	47	70	81	71	78	77	90	59	70	$1.10	800-365-1334
57	59	60	48	33	26	84	84	84	49	64	66	–	–	76	90	48	–	–	800-832-3211
75	81	82	74	60	51	92	95	94	58	68	77	–	–	75	89	62	–	–	800-538-5038
79	86	84	56	44	35	82	93	91	52	70	79	–	–	77	92	45	–	–	800-624-6519
60	75	79	71	56	60	89	88	94	43	–	–	–	–	–	–	–	–	–	800-538-5038
76	75	69	66	46	38	83	84	78	61	68	79	–	–	76	91	48	–	–	801-942-6200
–	–	–	–	–	–	–	–	–	–	72	82	–	–	80	93	57	–	–	801-741-8900
–	–	–	–	–	–	–	–	–	–	79	76	82	83	86	94	54	74	–	800-247-2583
–	–	–	–	–	–	–	–	–	–	74	73	74	84	85	92	71	88	–	888-888-4742
51	61	52	40	26	21	80	81	79	30	–	–	–	–	–	–	–	–	–	800-331-0150
–	–	–	–	–	–	–	–	–	–	78	76	76	85	86	94	72	87	$1.47	888-687-6277
–	–	–	–	–	–	–	–	–	–	76	73	76	82	85	93	64	80	–	800-247-2583
39	38	41	29	20	18	62	66	75	351	68	71	74	76	76	89	60	74	$1.08	800-323-9930
62	62	59	44	37	33	78	81	82	305	71	72	77	80	77	87	65	80	$1.02	800-296-5555
50	50	45	31	28	21	65	68	72	254	64	68	72	74	76	88	65	76	–	800-832-3211
–	–	–	–	–	–	–	–	–	–	74	75	79	80	78	91	68	86	–	800-832-3211
40	42	40	28	18	16	57	63	72	79	68	74	77	80	76	89	67	88	$0.96	800-304-0372
–	–	–	–	–	–	–	–	–	–	81	79	81	89	86	93	72	92	–	800-224-6599
53	52	64	55	48	46	60	64	77	179	63	73	64	78	77	85	74	64	$0.86	800-777-7902
50	49	51	34	31	25	69	73	73	319	73	71	75	84	78	90	75	87	$0.96	800-782-1966
77	80	71	57	32	36	91	84	88	25	77	78	80	–	81	91	78	91	$1.12	757-552-7401
77	80	71	57	32	36	91	84	88	25	76	79	80	–	81	91	77	93	$1.12	757-552-7401

Accreditation status with NCQA (1/2002) is shown. Accreditation status with JCAHO (1/2002) is shown as follows: JCAHO=With commendation or with full standards compliance; JCAHO=With requirements for improvement. **Accreditation with the American **Accreditation HealthCare Commission is shown as: AAHC.** None=No accreditation action reported by any of the three accrediting organizations.

Plan Ratings

✓ means plan receives our top rating

Highest scores are in Blue

Lowest scores are in *Bold Italic*

"–" means no data

Footnotes are on page 56

	Doctors' overall rating of plan for patient care (% favorable)	Members' overall rating of plan (% favorable)	Direct measures of actual care for which plan was among the best or worst plans (see codes below)*		Accreditation status**	% of members who had a problem (lower is better)	
			Best	Worst or not reported		"Big" problem getting referrals/tests/care	Called/wrote plan with complaint or problem
Average for all plans	57	60				9	20
Virginia (continued)							
Optimum Choice (All or most of Virginia)	54	62	b	f	Excellent	9	16
PARTNERS Nat'l HP of NC[2] (Blacksburg, Danville, Lynch., Roanoke)	55	62	deghi	j	Excellent	9	22
Peninsula Health Care (All or most of Virginia)	–	57	None	agj	Excellent	8	14
Priority Health Care (Most of Virginia)	51	64	cfk	a	Excellent	7	13
Southern Hlth Svcs (Danville, Fredericksburg, Richmond, Roanoke)	–	65	b	k	Commendable	6	19
UnitedHealthcare of the Mid-Atlantic (HMO) (Northern Virginia)	57	*54*	–	–	JCAHO	5	*25*
Washington							
Aetna U.S. Healthcare (Puget Sound area)	55	*50*	dej	gh	None	*13*	21
✓ Group Health Cooperative (HMO) (Most of Washington)	71	60	aceijk	b	Excellent	10	9
Group Health Options (Most of Washington)	–	57	aceijk	None	None	10	17
Group Health Options (POS) (Most of Washington)	–	*53*	cgk	bh	None	10	18
Health Net Health Plan of Oregon[20] (Southeastern Washington)	47	–	–	–	None	–	–
✓ Kaiser Permanente Northwest (HMO) (Southwestern Washington)	78	62	abcfgik	None	Excellent	*11*	11
✓ KPS Health Plans (HMO) (Puget Sound area)	–	82	–	–	None	1	15
PacifiCare of Oregon (HMO) (Southwestern Washington)	47	*54*	i	ch	Excellent	*13*	18
PacifiCare of WA (HMO) (Puget Sound area and most of western WA)	–	*52*	None	bcgh	Excellent	*13*	22
✓ Premera Blue Cross (All or most of Washington)	73	57	dij	bch	Excellent	9	17
✓ Providence Health Plans (Southwestern Washington)	73	60	di	h	Excellent	10	17
Regence HMO Oregon (Southwestern Washington)	79	*50*	k	abcghij	Commendable	–	–
RegenceCare (Seattle area)	73	–	–	–	None	–	–
West Virginia							
CIGNA HealthCare Mid-Atlantic (Beckley and Morgan counties)	50	*48*	bch	i	Excellent	*13*	22
✓ The Health Plan of the Upper Ohio Valley (HMO) (No.-central/NW WV)	–	77	de	bcfghij	Excellent	–	–
✓ HealthAmerica (HMO) (Northern West Virginia)	52	74	abdefghik	None	Excellent	6	17
HealthAmerica (POS) (Northern West Virginia)	52	60	abdfghik	None	Excellent	6	17
Optimum Choice (All or most of West Virginia)	54	62	b	f	Excellent	9	16
Wisconsin							
CompcareBlue (All or most of Wisconsin)	67	*51*	cij	fgh	None	8	*32*
✓ Dean Health Plan (HMO) (Southern Wisconsin)	–	72	acdegij	h	Excellent	6	12
✓ Group Health Cooperative of Eau Claire (HMO) (Eau Claire area)	–	79	dehij	bg	None	5	12
✓ Group Health Cooperative of South Central WI (HMO) (Madison area)	–	70	acdegij	None	Excellent	7	9
✓ Gunderson Lutheran Health Plan (HMO) (Southwestern Wisconsin)	–	73	–	–	None	5	14

*Assuring proper prevention and screening: a=Adolescent immunizations; b=Childhood immunizations; c=Chlamydia screening in sexually active women; d=Breast cancer screening; e=Cervical cancer screening. Assuring proper treatment: f=Beta blocker treatment after a heart attack; g=Cholesterol management (two measures); h=Controlling high blood pressure; i=Comprehensive diabetes care (six measures); j=Use of appropriate asthma medication; k=Followup after hospitalization for mental illness. "Best" or "worst" indicates plan's scores were in either the top or bottom 25 percent of benchmark plans.

Detailed performance measures

Ratings by doctors (% favorable)										Ratings by members (% favorable)									
Ability of patients to see appropriate specialists	Ability of patients to get needed tests and treatments	Ability of patients to get appropriate drugs	Plan's programs to help doctors give better care	How plan helps doctors follow up with patients	Incentives plan gives doctors affecting quality of care	Quality of primary care physicians affiliated with plan	Quality of specialists affiliated with plan	Quality of hospitals doctors can refer to within the plan	Number of doctors rating plan on the survey	Overall health care	Personal doctors	Specialist doctors	No problem getting referrals/tests/care	Getting care quickly	How well doctors communicate	Plan's customer service	Plan's claims processing	Estimated cost index for single person	Plan's phone number
56	56	52	42	36	30	72	76	78		73	75	77	79	78	90	67	81	$1.00	800-999-9999
54	51	52	37	32	26	72	76	76	314	69	68	77	79	75	88	70	83	–	800-331-2102
47	57	47	37	34	31	76	81	80	145	76	78	81	80	82	92	68	82	–	800-942-5695
–	–	–	–	–	–	–	–	–	–	69	72	74	84	78	90	69	90	–	800-304-0372
44	42	32	25	15	18	62	67	64	41	71	78	79	85	79	91	77	92	–	800-304-0372
–	–	–	–	–	–	–	–	–	–	78	79	78	85	80	92	70	84	–	800-627-4872
63	60	49	35	29	25	67	73	78	223	73	78	77	84	77	89	57	71	–	800-368-1680
58	63	63	46	31	27	80	83	85	102	71	72	79	72	80	91	62	75	$0.94	800-323-9930
66	63	67	78	60	47	79	79	78	59	69	72	73	80	81	90	72	84	$1.04[5]	888-901-4636
–	–	–	–	–	–	–	–	–	–	71	70	75	80	81	90	67	75	–	800-542-6312
–	–	–	–	–	–	–	–	–	–	68	71	73	78	79	92	66	77	–	800-542-6312
54	55	50	33	26	18	80	81	88	85	–	–	–	–	–	–	–	–	–	503-802-7000
71	74	85	81	71	66	85	83	76	55	69	76	72	81	77	89	77	84	$1.05	800-813-2000
–	–	–	–	–	–	–	–	–	–	87	83	85	94	90	94	77	94	$1.52	800-628-3753
39	43	48	34	26	22	73	82	89	106	66	68	76	72	76	89	63	89	$1.29	800-932-3004
–	–	–	–	–	–	–	–	–	–	74	72	80	72	83	90	60	78	$1.29	800-932-3004
69	69	63	53	37	29	85	90	87	95	73	72	78	80	83	92	65	85	–	800-691-3072
66	72	71	56	52	35	92	94	90	110	68	69	76	77	79	86	68	88	–	800-878-4445
77	78	73	57	48	39	92	93	92	114	71	72	79	–	82	92	60	85	–	800-228-0978
67	68	61	48	35	28	89	86	85	95	–	–	–	–	–	–	–	–	–	800-222-6129
50	50	45	31	28	21	65	68	72	254	64	68	72	74	76	88	65	76	–	800-832-3211
–	–	–	–	–	–	–	–	–	–	84	80	88	–	85	94	82	96	$0.98	800-624-6961
52	46	33	32	26	19	80	81	77	68	82	78	79	86	85	93	72	87	$0.94	800-788-8445
52	46	33	32	26	19	80	81	77	68	82	77	82	86	84	93	67	79	–	800-788-8445
54	51	52	37	32	26	72	76	76	314	69	68	77	79	75	88	70	83	–	800-331-2102
69	64	59	53	38	35	87	88	90	58	75	78	78	82	85	92	55	70	–	800-472-5811
–	–	–	–	–	–	–	–	–	–	80	82	74	86	86	92	74	93	$0.98	800-279-1301
–	–	–	–	–	–	–	–	–	–	85	85	80	89	91	96	78	93	$1.39	888-203-7770
–	–	–	–	–	–	–	–	–	–	72	75	76	86	86	91	75	92	$0.95	608-251-3356
–	–	–	–	–	–	–	–	–	–	76	82	72	90	84	92	73	91	–	608-775-8000

Accreditation status with NCQA (1/2002) is shown. Accreditation status with JCAHO (1/2002) is shown as follows: JCAHO=With commendation or with full standards compliance; JCAHO=With requirements for improvement. **Accreditation with the American

Accreditation HealthCare Commission is shown as: AAHC. None=No accreditation action reported by any of the three accrediting organizations.

Plan Ratings

✓ means plan receives our top rating
Highest scores are in Blue
Lowest scores are in **_Bold Italic_**
"—" means no data

	Doctors' overall rating of plan for patient care (% favorable)	Members' overall rating of plan (% favorable)	Key performance measures		Accreditation status**	% of members who had a problem (lower is better)	
			Direct measures of actual care for which plan was among the best or worst plans (see codes below)*				
			Best	Worst or not reported		"Big" problem getting referrals/tests/care	Called/wrote plan with complaint or problem
Average for all plans	57	60				9	20
Wisconsin *(continued)*							
HMO Illinois/BlueAdvantage (HMO) (Kenosha County)	58	56	a	bchj	Excellent	**_11_**	23
Humana Wisconsin (HMO) (Southeastern Wisconsin)	**_31_**	55	ah	f	None	10	**_30_**
✓ Medica (Western Wisconsin)	72	64	None	g	Excellent	8	15
Medical Associates Health Plans (Southwestern Wisconsin)	—	69	d	abcghij	Commendable	—	—
Network Health Plan of Wisconsin (HMO) (Southeastern Wisconsin)	—	56	abcdegi	None	Commendable	10	16
Physicians Plus (Southern Wisconsin)	—	61	adefhijk	b	Excellent	8	14
✓ Security Health Plan (HMO) (Northern, western, and central Wisconsin)	—	71	adefgijk	None	None	4	7
✓ Touchpoint Health Plan (HMO) (Northeastern Wisconsin)	—	67	abdefgijk	None	Excellent	5	13
Touchpoint Health Plan (POS) (Northeastern Wisconsin)	—	**_51_**	acdeik	None	Excellent	10	20
✓ UnitedHealthcare of Wisconsin (Southeastern Wisconsin)	74	68	ack	f	Excellent	5	16
Unity Health Plans (Southwestern and south-central Wisconsin)	—	65	acdeghijk	b	None	7	17
✓ Valley Health Plan (Western Wisconsin)	—	79	dgijk	None	Accredited	5	9
Wyoming							
Intermountain Health Care (Parts of Western Wyoming)	93	61	—	—	Commendable	—	—

*Assuring proper prevention and screening: a=Adolescent immunizations; b=Childhood immunizations; c=Chlamydia screening in sexually active women; d=Breast cancer screening; e=Cervical cancer screening. **Assuring proper treatment:** f=Beta blocker treatment after a heart attack; g=Cholesterol management (two measures); h=Controlling high blood pressure; i=Comprehensive diabetes care (six measures); j=Use of appropriate asthma medication; k=Followup after hospitalization for mental illness. "Best" or "worst" indicates plan's scores were in either the top or bottom 25 percent of benchmark plans.

Footnotes

[1] Formerly PHS.

[2] Plan changed ownership during survey periods; management policies may have changed.

[3] Plan is also accredited by JCAHO (accredited with full standards compliance).

[4] Member satisfaction data for this plan were collected using a questionnaire and a data collection protocol that were slightly different from what was used for other plans. It is possible that the plan scored slightly better or worse than it would have if the standard questionnaire and protocol had been used.

[5] Cost data reported are based on plan's cost structure for the Seattle area.

[6] Costs data reported are based on plan's cost structure for the northern Ohio area.

[7] Formerly Health Net.

[8] Plan is also accredited by AAHC.

[9] Cost data reported are based on plan's cost structure for the Detroit area.

[10] Formerly Empire Health Care.

[11] Plan is also accredited by JCAHO (accredited with commendation).

[11] Plan is also accredited by JCAHO (accredited with requirements for improvement).

[13] Cost data reported are based on plan's cost structure for the Downstate New York area.

[14] Cost data reported are based on plan's cost structure for the Albany area.

[15] Formerly EmpireHealth Choice.

[16] Cost data reported are based on plan's cost structure for New York City.

[17] Cost data reported are based on plan's cost structure for the Central New York area.

[18] Formerly Healthsource.

[19] The information available for analysis for this plan included only eight of the 11 measures—not the chlamydia screening, blood pressure, or asthma measures—so the plan could not score either favorably or unfavorably on more than eight measures.

[20] Formerly QualMed.

[21] Formerly Physicians Health Plan.

[22] The information available for analysis for this plan included only eight of the 11 measures—not the adolescent immunization, beta blocker treatment, or cholesterol management measures—so the plan could not score either favorably or unfavorably on more than eight measures.

Detailed performance measures																			
Ratings by doctors (% favorable)											Ratings by members (% favorable)								
Ability of patients to see appropriate specialists	Ability of patients to get needed tests and treatments	Ability of patients to get appropriate drugs	Plan's programs to help doctors give better care	How plan helps doctors follow up with patients	Incentives plan gives doctors affecting quality of care	Quality of primary care physicians affiliated with plan	Quality of specialists affiliated with plan	Quality of hospitals doctors can refer to within the plan	Number of doctors rating plan on the survey	Overall health care	Personal doctors	Specialist doctors	No problem getting referrals/tests/care	Getting care quickly	How well doctors communicate	Plan's customer service	Plan's claims processing	Estimated cost index for single person	Plan's phone number
56	56	52	42	36	30	72	76	78		73	75	77	79	78	90	67	81	$1.00	800-999-9999
54	54	55	46	39	35	74	76	76	189	68	71	66	76	76	88	62	70	–	800-892-2803
33	38	29	29	22	9	72	78	71	55	74	76	77	77	83	92	58	73	–	800-448-6262
74	75	62	49	36	34	89	95	91	206	80	83	81	85	80	92	69	86	–	800-952-3455
–	–	–	–	–	–	–	–	–	–	74	78	77	–	84	91	74	91	–	800-747-8900
–	–	–	–	–	–	–	–	–	–	61	65	71	80	72	88	70	89	–	920-720-1452
–	–	–	–	–	–	–	–	–	–	75	79	74	84	80	92	63	87	–	800-545-5015
–	–	–	–	–	–	–	–	–	–	80	83	81	91	88	94	80	95	–	800-472-2363
–	–	–	–	–	–	–	–	–	–	77	74	78	88	85	93	76	92	–	800-441-4469
–	–	–	–	–	–	–	–	–	–	71	68	76	79	81	91	64	78	–	800-441-4469
74	71	67	58	47	40	85	89	81	54	75	76	73	89	85	91	74	92	–	800-407-3776
–	–	–	–	–	–	–	–	–	–	77	78	74	86	83	92	68	90	$1.11	800-362-3310
–	–	–	–	–	–	–	–	–	–	85	86	80	91	90	96	80	96	–	800-472-5411
75	81	82	74	60	51	92	95	94	58	68	77	–	–	75	89	62	–	–	800-538-5038

Accreditation status with NCQA (1/2002) is shown. Accreditation status with JCAHO (1/2002) is shown as follows: JCAHO=With commendation or with full standards compliance; JCAHO=With requirements for improvement. **Accreditation with the American**

Accreditation HealthCare Commission is shown as: AAHC. None=No accreditation action reported by any of the three accrediting organizations.

Chapter 5

Choosing a Plan: Finding Low Costs and Good Coverage

F inding a plan that offers high-quality care and good service is only part of the battle. You also want to keep your costs down.

You want not just low premiums but also broad coverage. The broader the coverage, the lower your out-of-pocket costs will be. You'll want to consider what you'll have to pay out-of-pocket in a good year in which you use very few medical services and in a bad year in which you are hospitalized and use extensive medical services.

You will be interested in premiums and coverage whether you are considering an HMO, a PPO, or a traditional indemnity plan. Premiums and coverage are the main considerations when choosing an indemnity plan because the quality differences among indemnity plans are relatively small—since those plans have very little control over the quality of service you receive from the doctors *you* choose.

Premiums

A first step in shopping for low costs is to get premium quotes from several plans. An independent agent can assist you by shopping a number of plans and presenting proposals to you for the plan or plans he or she thinks best fit your needs. But there are some companies—for example, State Farm and some HMOs—that sell plans only through their own employees or their own agents. To include such plans among your

options, you'll have to call representatives of these companies. In addition, it's a good idea, if you are doing the shopping for your employer or if you are self-employed, to find out whether there are trade associations that sponsor plans for firms in your industry and get quotes from any appropriate association.

There are many websites that offer rate quotes. In many cases, these are just agents or brokers who will use the website to collect information from you and eventually send you back some quotes. Some of these sites have information forms that will help you put down in one place the pertinent facts; you might want to do this and then send the factsheet to agents or companies of your choice. There are a few websites that give you immediate quotes and plan/benefit descriptions online. That at least gives you a reference point, but keep in mind that these sites generally list only plans with which they do business, often not the best available plans.

Many factors affect rates. With most, but not all plans, age is important. For example, in one plan we checked, the annual premium cost was more than four times higher for a 57-year-old single male than for a 27-year-old single male. If you are over 50 or shopping for an employer group made up of older employees, a plan that doesn't set premiums based on age may be an especially good bargain.

Gender is also an important factor, especially among plans that offer maternity benefits. For example, the annual premium cost we found in one plan for a single, 27-year-old female was more than twice the cost for a single male the same age. But a number of plans—even some that include maternity coverage—set rates without regard to gender.

A third important consideration is location. For example, one California plan we checked charged about 10 percent more for someone in San Francisco than for a person across the San Francisco Bay in Contra Costa County. Generally, employment-based group plans look to the location of the business, and plans that are sold to individuals look to the individual's residence. Different plans have different geographic adjustment factors and define rate territories in different ways. Some may treat a large metropolitan area as a single territory, while others will have different rates for each county or Zip Code.

Even for groups or individuals of the exact same age and gender, in the same region, some plans have much higher premiums than others. For example, for a 47-year-old female, one California plan we checked was charging $3,700 per year, while another with similar benefits was charging only $1,270. That's a difference of more than $2,400.

There are many reasons that some plans charge more than others for the same individual or group. Some of these reasons have nothing to do with the quality of the plan from your point of view as an enrollee. For example, a plan's premiums may be high because the plan has attracted a relatively unhealthy, high-cost pool of enrollees over the years. A plan might have such a pool because it offers some benefit feature that makes

About the Cost Index Scores...

On the Plan Ratings table in Chapter 4, you will find cost index scores for many of the plans. These are the plans that participate in the health insurance program for Federal employees. The cost index score for each plan shows how the plan compared to the other rated plans according to our estimate of premiums plus likely out-of-pocket costs for an average single enrollee. The index scores are set so that the average is $1.00. A plan with an index score of, for example, $1.20 is estimated to be 20 percent more costly than average for premiums and out-of-pocket costs. For a number of reasons, this is only an extremely rough reference point for looking at costs even among the plans for which we have an index. For example, it will not be of use if a plan has a healthier mix of members, relative to other plans, in your geographic area or group compared to its mix in the Federal employee program. And it doesn't take into account how your personal cost will be affected if your employer pays a portion of premiums.

it attractive to "high-risk" groups; for instance, plans that offer extensive psychiatric benefits have tended to attract relatively high-cost enrollees. Also, some plans might use a marketing approach that brings in disproportionate numbers of unhealthy customers, or they might use relatively lax standards in accepting new customers. Whatever the cause, a plan that has a high-cost pool of enrollees has to raise premiums high enough to pay claims.

Although cost differences among plans often have nothing to do with quality, sometimes they do. For example, some plans have relatively low premiums because they offer fewer benefits than others offer, some have stringent policies that make it difficult to get claims paid, and some HMO plans may include relatively low-quality doctors or be restrictive in the care they authorize. The table below shows that among HMOs—where the plan has a lot to do with the actual quality of care you receive—higher cost plans (considering both premiums and out-of-pocket costs for services not covered by benefits) tend to get better ratings from physicians and to have more satisfied customers, although they are less likely to be accredited, than lower cost plans. Fortunately, there are many lower cost plans that rate very high on all quality measures.

Do You Get What You Pay For?

	Average percent of physicians who rated plan "good," "very good," or "excellent"	Average percent of members who rated the overall care of plan "8" or better on a 0 to 10 scale	Percent of plans that are accredited
Lowest cost one-third of plans	47%	59%	90%
Medium cost one-third of plans	53%	63%	85%
Highest cost one-third of plans	57%	64%	61%

Plans were divided into three groups based on premium plus estimated out-of-pocket costs for a single federal government employee. Table includes data for the 124 plans on the "Plan Ratings" table that participate in the Federal Employees Health Benefits Program.

Benefits

In comparing benefits, you'll want to check several questions. The worksheet on pages 62 and 63 will help. You'll find less variation among HMOs than among indemnity plans and PPOs.

What Types of Services Are Covered?

Most plans pick up some portion of the cost of hospitals, physicians, and prescription drugs. Some also make a contribution to the costs of skilled nursing homes, home health care services, hospice care, and mental health services in or out of a hospital. A few cover additional services—such as dental care or vision care—usually as an extra-cost option. Particular details may be of special importance to you—such as coverage of chiropractors; acupuncturists; Christian Science practitioners; physical, speech, or occupational therapists; and various types of products ranging from prosthetic devices to blood supplies to insulin.

You must be careful to note the exact limits of coverage. For example, plans may pay different portions (or none at all) of the costs of services depending on whether the services are surgical as opposed to medical,

delivered inside a hospital as opposed to a doctor's office, for treatment of a medical problem as opposed to a preventive checkup, or related to an emergency as opposed to a nonemergency. Some of the lowest cost plans, in fact, pay only for services that are delivered while the enrollee is an inpatient in a hospital.

Also, plans sometimes pay differently, or not at all, depending on the specific conditions being treated. A plan that excludes from coverage, for example, the costs of routine pregnancy may be an acceptable choice for you if you and your dependents are unlikely to become pregnant or can handle the predictable costs of a pregnancy. But you won't want to consider plans that cover only cancer and certain other "dread diseases" since you can't anticipate whether other equally costly medical problems might occur.

How Is the Level of Covered Charges Figured?

For any given type of service—say, inpatient services of a surgeon—plans set limits on the level of charges they will allow. The insurance company simply won't pay a fee that it considers too high. Unfortunately, such limits may leave the patient to make up the difference if a plan's concept of what is too high is different from the service provider's concept.

Many plans promise to pay "usual, customary, and reasonable" (UCR) charges. Some plans provide no definition of such terms. Even where a definition is provided, it may leave questions unanswered. For example, one indemnity policy we examined defined the UCR limit in its plan as the lesser of: (1) the fee most often charged by the provider; (2) the fee most often charged in the locality where the service was performed; or (3) the fee which is recognized as reasonable by a prudent person.

What does "most often charged in the locality" mean? Does it include a surgeon's fee if the fee is higher than that charged by the lowest priced 50 percent of the locality's other surgeons? What if the surgeon's fee is higher than that charged by 60 percent—or 80 percent—of the locality's other surgeons? Also, how broadly is "locality" defined, and are allowances made for a surgeon's special expertise? Similar questions arise when plans say they'll pay "prevailing" charges or simply "reasonable" charges. Even if a plan ultimately pays or if a provider eventually agrees to adjust a fee, a lot of time may be spent getting to the resolution.

Unfortunately, there's no easy way for you to find out in advance just how reasonable a plan's standards will be. All you can do is press for as precise a definition of the standards as possible, ask an independent agent who has regularly dealt with the plan how satisfied his or her clients have been, and, perhaps, talk directly with some persons the plan currently insures.

Although imprecise standards can be a problem, greater concerns are raised by plans that allow charges only up to a "fee schedule" that they have established. If such a plan's fee schedule says it will allow a maximum surgeon's fee of $600 for an appendectomy and your surgeon in fact charges $1,200, you have to pick up the entire $600 difference.

Often it is difficult, when comparing plans, to find out details of a plan's fee schedule, and even if you can get the information, it will be difficult for you to judge how generous the schedule is.

The safest arrangement, with regard to the level of covered charges, is a policy that simply covers the full amount that is billed. PPOs and HMOs offer such coverage for charges by participating providers—because they negotiate with each provider in advance the maximum that the provider will charge (or, in the case of some HMOs, because the providers are on salary).

What Deductible Must You Pay Before the Plan Starts Paying?

Most non-HMO plans require each enrollee to pay a certain amount— a "deductible"—out-of-pocket before the plan begins paying. A typical plan might require the enrollee to pay the first $250 in covered charges, but deductible requirements range from zero to several thousand dollars. Many plans allow each individual policyholder or employment-based group to select from among several deductible levels, with lower premiums resulting from higher deductibles.

In addition to checking the size of the deductible, find out how many deductibles a family must satisfy. A plan that has a $250 deductible per person, for example, might begin to pay claims for all family members as soon as the family has paid $250 out-of-pocket for two family members even if the other family members haven't met their deductibles.

Many plans allow enrollees to count toward a year's deductible the expenses that could have been charged toward the deductible in the last three months of the previous year.

Some plans add on an extra deductible if you fail to meet certain conditions—for example, if you neglect to get approval from the plan before having surgery. On the other hand, some plans waive deductibles if you meet specified conditions—for example, if you use a "preferred provider" or if you have surgery done in an outpatient clinic rather than incurring the expense of treatment as an overnight patient in a hospital.

What Percent of Covered Charges Is Paid?

Most non-HMO plans pay only a portion of each covered expense and expect the enrollee to pay the rest. A typical setup is for the plan to pay 80 percent and the enrollee 20 percent. But you can select a plan that pays as much as 100 percent or as little as 50 percent. In many cases, the percentage a plan pays— referred to as its share of "coinsurance"—is higher for some types of services than for others—for example, outpatient surgery versus inpatient surgery, or mental health services versus medical services— and in many cases PPOs pay a higher percentage for services performed by "preferred" providers than for services performed by others.

Some HMO and PPO plans expect the enrollee to pay a fixed dollar amount—called a "copayment"— for each unit of service. For instance, the enrollee might pay $10 per physician's office visit rather than a percentage of the doctor's charge.

How Using a PPO's Providers Can Save You Money

It is important to note that using a PPO's preferred providers can save you money in two ways—compared to going outside the PPO's provider list or compared to using a traditional indemnity plan. The figure on the right illustrates the savings. First, by using a PPO's doctors, you avoid paying any portion of the provider's regular fee that exceeds the PPO's approved fee schedule; the PPO providers have agreed to limit their fees for PPO members to the PPO's approved maximum. Second, when you use a PPO provider, the plan generally pays a higher percentage of the approved fee than when you use other providers.

What Is the Maximum Out-of-Pocket Expense?

Many plans set a maximum on the amount the enrollee will have to pay out-of-pocket for covered expenses. Common limits are $1,000 or $2,500 per family member. With many plans, the enrollee's out-of-pocket expense for the deductible is not counted toward the stated out-of-pocket limit. Here's how an out-of-pocket limit might work for a plan with a $250 deductible, 80 percent coinsurance, and $1,000 out-of-pocket limit. Suppose an enrollee had surgery with total covered expenses equal to $10,000. The enrollee would pay the first $250 as a deductible, then would pay 20 percent of the next $5,000. The plan would pay 80 percent of the $5,000 between $250 and $5,250 and would pay 100 percent of the amount above $5,250. The total cost to the enrollee would be $1,250 ($1,000 coinsurance plus $250 deductible), and the cost to the plan would be $8,750 (its $4,000 share of coinsurance and all charges above $5,250).

Some plans have a separate out-of-pocket limit for each family member; others have a single limit for the entire family. Some plans state their limits not as the maximum the enrollee will have to pay but rather as the amount the plan has to pay out before the enrollee can stop contributing.

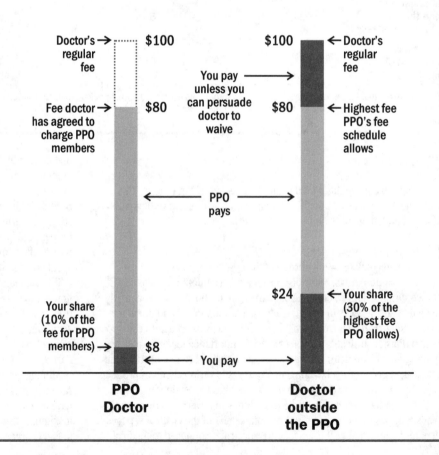

The Extra Cost When a PPO Member Uses a Non-PPO Doctor

An out-of-pocket limit is very important: it protects you from financial catastrophe. But check the details carefully. Often charges for certain services—such as mental health services or nursing home care—aren't counted toward the limit. And no plan will count toward its limit costs that result from fees in excess of its fee schedule or "usual, customary, and reasonable" standard.

Are There Other Limits on Benefits?

For specific types of services, you may find specific limits. Many plans limit the number of nursing home days, for example, or the number of home health care visits or outpatient mental health visits or hospital days. Also, some limit the total amount they will pay—say, a maximum of $5,000 per year and $25,000 in a lifetime for mental health services.

What Is the Minimum Package of Benefits That Meets Your Needs?

Don't pay for any benefits that you don't need. You save substantial amounts by eliminating benefits you feel sure won't be used. For example, in one popular plan we checked, dropping maternity coverage in a policy for a 25-year-old male employee with spouse and one child would save $1,045 per year.

Remember that the function of insurance is to protect against catastrophe—not to pay everyday expenses. Consider your financial resources (or the resources of each member of your employee group if you are shopping for an employer). How much health care expense can be absorbed without serious disruption? Will you be able to borrow (or are there loan programs an employer offers or can set up) so that expenses can be spread over a period of time?

By selecting the lowest acceptable insurance company coinsurance percentage and the highest acceptable deductible and out-of-pocket limit, you'll cut premiums significantly. For example, in one plan we checked, starting with a $250 deductible and $1,000 out-of-pocket maximum, the annual premium cost for a 35-year-old male employee with spouse and child was $3,300 with 80 percent coinsurance, but was $2,700 if the coinsurance level was changed to 50 percent. Raising the deductible resulted in further reductions to $2,500 with a $500 deductible, or $2,200 with a $1,000 deductible. Total savings for this enrollee was $1,100 while still limiting the enrollee's financial exposure to a possible $1,000 out-of-pocket for coinsurance and a $1,000 deductible.

Although this plan did not allow the option of increasing the out-of-pocket limit, many plans do. Going from a $1,000 limit to a $2,500 limit might reduce the premium by five percent or more.

Other Plan Features

In addition to premiums and benefits, there are other important plan features affecting the breadth and soundness of coverage—and the likelihood that you'll be able to get coverage at all. Some of these features are considerations only if you are shopping for an employer, not if you are looking for an individual plan.

Cost Containment Provisions

Many insurance policies have provisions designed to assure that services are used only after careful consideration of whether they are necessary and whether less expensive alternatives would achieve comparable results.

Plans have always reserved the right to refuse to pay for services that are "not medically necessary," but it is difficult for a plan to make that determination after the service has been rendered. A plan's refusal to pay at that time is a very harsh blow to the enrollee who must pay from his or her own pocket or to the provider who must do without payment. Special cost containment provisions move forward the decision regarding medical necessity and appropriateness. The most common provisions require the enrollee to seek approval from the plan prior to hospital admission and prior to extending a hospital stay beyond the originally approved duration, and require the enrollee to get a second professional opinion before certain surgery.

These provisions are intended to encourage a dialogue from which there may emerge agreement that a procedure simply isn't appropriate or that it can be done in a less costly setting—outpatient rather than inpatient surgery, for example, or home health care rather than an extension of time in the hospital.

Some plans "require" enrollees to follow cost containment procedures but impose no sanctions other than the risk of later disapproval of charges as "unnecessary" if the procedures aren't followed. Others increase deductibles or coinsurance requirements for treatments that aren't preceded by proper cost containment procedures—even if these treatments are determined to be entirely appropriate.

Preexisting Condition Limitations

Another way for plans to hold down costs is to exclude from coverage "preexisting conditions."

For individuals and small groups, insurance companies typically require submission of a medical history, reporting on previous illnesses, hospitalizations, and doctor visits. Reporting usually covers the previous five years or more. The insurer can independently check much of the health-history information using industry data-banks.

Typically, insurance companies have a blanket "preexisting" condition exclusion that applies to all individual enrollees or group members. A company might, for instance, exclude from coverage "any condition for which a person received any medical attention, consultation, or treatment or for which distinct symptoms were evident six months prior to the effective date of insurance." By excluding such conditions, a plan spares itself the cost of treating them, of course, and perhaps more important, it avoids attracting individuals or groups with members who may tend to be relatively illness-prone.

There are three separate aspects of most of these blanket provisions regarding preexisting conditions—

- How many prior months are considered in determining whether a condition should be counted as a preexisting condition;
- How many months under the plan qualify an enrollee for full coverage of a preexisting condition if the enrollee requires no treatment during the period; and
- How many months under the plan qualify the enrollee for full coverage if the enrollee requires continuing treatment during the period.

In addition to blanket provisions regarding preexisting conditions, insurance companies sometimes specifically exclude from coverage certain conditions of a specific enrollee, based on the enrollee's detailed medical history. The insurance company may look back into the history several years and may issue a policy with a "rider" that excludes coverage for a long time or permanently. This kind of insurance company determination is an element of what is referred to as underwriting. Depending on the number and types of preexisting conditions an individual applicant has, or a group's members have, an insurance company may refuse to cover, or may impose an extra premium surcharge on, the individual applicant, specific group members, or an entire group.

(Text continues on page 64)

Coverage and Features Comparison Worksheet

	PPO Illustration		HMO Illustration
Company name	Sample Insurance Company		Sample HMO Company
Plan name	Sample PPO Plan		Sample HMO Plan
Minimum group size	2		5
Provider type	Preferred providers	Nonpreferred providers	HMO providers
Annual deductible per person	$250	$250	None
How many deductibles per family	3	3	N/A
How much company pays for...			
Hospital room and board	80 percent	60 percent	100 percent
Other hospital-billed inpatient supplies and services	80 percent	60 percent	100 percent
Inpatient surgical services	80 percent	60 percent	100 percent
Other inpatient doctor services	80 percent	60 percent	100 percent
Outpatient hospital supplies and services	80 percent	60 percent	100 percent
Outpatient surgical services	80 percent	60 percent	100 percent after $10/visit
Other outpatient doctor services	80 percent	60 percent	100 percent after $10/visit
Outpatient diagnostic tests	80 percent	60 percent	100 percent after $10/visit
Prescription drugs	100 percent after copayment of $10 generic, $25 brand name	100 percent of plan's limited fee schedule after copay. of $10 generic, $25 brand name	100 percent after $10 copayment
How level of covered charges is figured	Negotiated fee—provider can't bill more	"Reasonable and customary"—you must pay all costs above this level	Negotiated fee—provider can't bill more
Max. annual out-of-pocket costs for hospital, doctor, and drugs, per person	$2,000/$4,000 plus deductibles	$2,000/$4,000 plus deductibles and amounts above "reasonable and customary"	No specific limit but most charges covered if plan providers used
Other services:			
Normal pregnancy	Option to cover same as other conditions	Option to cover same as other conditions	Covered same as other conditions
Inpatient care for mental and nervous disorders	50 percent of negotiated fee up to $5,000 per year	50 percent of "reasonable" charges up to $5,000 per year	100 percent up to 30 days per year
Outpatient care for mental and nervous disorders	50 percent of negotiated fee, but no more than $25/visit up to $5,000 per year	50 percent of "reasonable" charges, but no more than $25/visit up to $5,000 per year	100 percent after $25/visit up to 20 visits per year
Routine checkups	Not covered	Not covered	Covered same as other doctor visits
Skilled nursing homes	60 percent of "reasonable and customary"	60 percent of "reasonable and customary"	100 percent up to 30 days per year
Home health care	60 percent of "reasonable and customary"	60 percent of "reasonable and customary"	100 percent
Other features: Cost containment features	$250 extra deductible if hospital admission not preapproved	$250 extra deductible if hospital admission not preapproved	All hospital stays and specialist services covered only if authorized by primary doctor
Preexisting conditions: How many prior months considered	12 months	12 months	No preexisting condition exclusion
How soon covered if treatment-free	6 months	6 months	N/A
How soon covered if not treatment-free	12 months	12 months	N/A
Are preexisting condition limits waived if plan takes over from previous plan?	Yes	Yes	N/A
What percent of employees must be in plan	100 percent in groups of 2 to 9; 80 percent in larger groups	100 percent in groups of 2 to 9; 80 percent in larger groups	5 employees (percent doesn't matter)
How much employer must contribute to premium	75 percent of employee costs or 50 percent of employee plus dependents	75 percent of employee costs or 50 percent of employee plus dependents	100 percent of employee cost
Hours/week employee must work to be eligible	30	30	20
Life insurance employee must buy	$15,000	$15,000	None
How long rate is guaranteed	6 months	6 months	12 months

	Your Plan Option 1	Your Plan Option 2
Company name		
Plan name		
Minimum group size		
Provider type		
Annual deductible per person		
How many deductibles per family		
How much company pays for...		
Hospital room and board		
Other hospital-billed inpatient supplies and services		
Inpatient surgical services		
Other inpatient doctor services		
Outpatient hospital supplies and services		
Outpatient surgical services		
Other outpatient doctor services		
Outpatient diagnostic tests		
Prescription drugs		
How level of covered charges is figured		
Max. annual out-of-pocket costs for hospital, doctor, and drugs, per person		
Other services:		
Normal pregnancy		
Inpatient care for mental and nervous disorders		
Outpatient care for mental and nervous disorders		
Routine checkups		
Skilled nursing homes		
Home health care		
Other features:		
Cost containment features		
Preexisting conditions: How many prior months considered		
How soon covered if treatment-free		
How soon covered if not treatment-free		
Are preexisting condition limits waived if plan takes over from previous plan?		
What percent of employees must be in plan		
How much employer must contribute to premium		
Hours/week employee must work to be eligible		
Life insurance employee must buy		
How long rate is guaranteed		

Many plans have special provisions regarding preexisting conditions when coverage is switched from one insurance company to another. Some group plans have "full takeover" of benefits, meaning that any conditions that would have been covered under the previous plan are covered under the new one.

Group Size

As we've noted, one way insurance companies avoid becoming burdened with a disproportionate number of high-risk enrollees is to insure groups rather than individuals. If only individuals are covered, there is the possibility that illness-prone individuals will seek coverage while healthier individuals take their chances without insurance or with bare-bones insurance. By covering a group, an insurance company enhances the chances that it will pick up at least some relatively healthy individuals. For this reason, many companies insure only large groups and others offer plans for small groups but not for individuals.

Although plans for employment-based groups are generally less expensive than plans open to individuals, there are exceptions. So an employer might want to consider buying an individual plan for each employee. Some insurance companies will arrange for a combined bill to simplify the employer's paperwork. Even if the cost of buying a package of individual plans in this way is somewhat higher than the cost of a group plan, the package of individual plans might be a better option because of "portability": if an employee leaves the company but picks up the cost of continued premium payments, the employee's coverage continues unchanged.

Requirements Regarding Participation, Employer Contribution, and Full-Time Employment

Plans that are available only to employment-based groups often impose several requirements to assure that they will get healthier employees along with those who are more illness-prone. Generally, group plans require that all or nearly all employees and dependents in a small group be insured (though there are often exceptions for spouses who are insured by another employer). To add to the incentive for full participation, they may also require that the employer contribute all or nearly all the premium at least for employees and possibly for both employees and dependents.

So that they won't be burdened with unhealthy individuals who are too sick to work full time or who work just a limited amount in order to qualify for a group health plan, most insurance companies limit enrollment to "full-time" employees. The definition of "full-time" may be someone who works as few as 17.5 hours per week or as high as 30 hours per week.

Industry Exclusions

Insurance companies often deny coverage to businesses in certain industries or to individual applicants in certain occupations. For example, some companies refuse to insure bars, restaurants, and beauty salons because rapid employee turnover results in high administrative costs. Also, high-risk industries such as mining or amusement park operation are often hard to insure. If you are an employer in a hard-to-insure business, or an individual applicant in a hard-to-insure occupation, your broker will have to shop widely for coverage. Sometimes a good broker can get coverage by persuading an insurance company to make an exception or to define the nature of your business or occupation as falling into an acceptable category. You should be sure also to check whether you can qualify for a plan offered by a business association or trade association in your industry.

Financial Soundness

If your insurance company goes out of business or discontinues offering your policy, you might have a risky period without coverage. Worse still, if you (or members of your group) have serious medical problems at the time, finding new coverage may be difficult.

There's no sure way to judge the staying power of an insurance company. But you can be reassured to a degree if the company has been selling policies of the type you're buying for a number of years and has a large number of enrollees. It is reassuring to know that a plan is offered by a number of large employers that would have the expertise to check out the plan's financial strength. In addition, you can ask your agent for the company's "Best" rating. A rating of "A+" or "A" is a favorable (but not sure-fire) indication of financial soundness. You can also find financial soundness ratings on most plans by calling Weiss Research at 1-800-289-9222 or by visiting *www.weissratings.com*. The fee per company is $15 by phone and $7.95 online.

Chapter 6

Choosing a Plan: Special Choices If You Are Eligible for Medicare

When you are eligible for Medicare, you have a different range of health insurance choices than other consumers have. In this chapter, which draws heavily on Federal government publications, we describe your Medicare benefits, identify gaps in your Medicare coverage, and give tips on choosing private health insurance to fill those gaps.

Various potential health care costs are not covered by Medicare. For example, you are responsible to pay a "deductible" amount before Medicare pays anything for a hospital stay, and Medicare does not pay at all for most prescription drugs.

If you have a serious disease or illness requiring extensive medical services, just covering the gaps in Medicare out of your own pocket can be financially ruinous. So many consumers rely on private insurance to cover some of the potential costs. There are several ways of extending your own coverage to fill in some of Medicare's gaps:

- *Purchase Medicare supplemental insurance*, also called "Medigap" or "MedSup" insurance. This can be traditional fee-for-service coverage, which provides the same level of coverage regardless of which doctors and other health care providers you use to deliver covered services. Or it can be a "SELECT" plan, which will cover a larger portion of your bill if you use the plan's pre-selected network of providers. If you have a Medigap policy, Medicare makes its usual payment for services and the Medigap plan pays all or part of what Medicare doesn't pay.
- *Enroll in a managed care plan*—a health maintenance organization (HMO), provider-sponsored organization (PSO), or preferred provider organization (PPO)—that has a contract to serve Medicare beneficiaries. With an HMO or PSO, your care may be covered only if you use providers in the plan's network; most specialist, laboratory, hospital, and other services are covered only if you are referred to them by your primary care doctor. Some HMO and PSO plans may have a point-of-service (POS) option, which allows you to use non-network providers if you are willing to pay higher out-of-pocket costs. With a PPO, you can use any provider without a referral, but you will have lower copayments or deductibles if you use a provider in the plan's network. (As of this writing, there were only two Medicare PPO plans, each serving only a limited geographic area.)
- *Continue coverage under an employer-provided health insurance policy, if your pre-retirement employer offers one.* Fewer and fewer employers offer such coverage to retirees. Those that do may offer fee-for-service options and various options that encourage or require you to use providers within an established network.
- *Select one of the options authorized under 1997 revisions to Medicare.* The revisions opened the market for fee-for-service plans. As of this writing, this option is available in limited areas of the U.S.

In addition to the information provided in this article on your options under Medicare, you can get information and advice from various senior citizen advocacy organizations and government agencies. All states now offer insurance counseling, at no charge to you, in one-on-one confidential sessions with trained counselors. In these sessions, you will be able to talk about insurance issues that you find confusing and get advice on your insurance needs. Telephone numbers and web addresses for the insurance counseling services in your area are listed in Appendix B.

The Centers for Medicare and Medicaid Services (CMS), the Federal agency that administers the Medicare program, has many publications and an increasingly useful website (*www.medicare.gov*) that will help you understand your Medicare options. A good starting point is the CMS publication, *Medicare & You 2002*, which is available from local Social Security offices or can be downloaded from the *www.medicare.gov* website.

Medicare Coverage and Gaps

Before considering Medigap coverage and the other types of private insurance available to supplement Medicare, it is helpful to review your Medicare benefits and identify the coverage gaps.

Medicare is a Federal health insurance program for persons 65 or older, persons of any age with permanent kidney failure, and certain disabled persons under 65. (In this article, we focus on the 65-and-over group; if you are in one of the other eligible categories, be sure to get advice from the Medicare insurance counseling service in your state.) CMS, which administers Medicare, is part of the U. S. Department of Health and Human Services (HHS). The Social Security Administration provides information about the program and handles enrollment.

Medicare has two parts—Hospital Insurance (Part A) and Medical Insurance (Part B). Part A is financed through part of the Social Security (FICA) tax paid by workers and their employers. You do not have to pay a monthly premium for Medicare Part A if you or your spouse is entitled to benefits under either the Social Security or Railroad Retirement systems or worked a sufficient period of time in Federal, state, or local government employment to be insured.

If you do not qualify for premium-free Part A benefits, you may purchase the coverage (for $319 per month in 2002, in most cases) if you are at least age 65 and meet certain requirements. Check with any Social Security office for details.

Part B is optional and is offered to all beneficiaries when they become entitled to Part A. It also may be purchased by most persons age 65 or over who do not qualify for premium-free Part A coverage. The Part B premium, which most Medicare beneficiaries have deducted from their monthly Social Security check, is $54 per month in 2002.

You are automatically enrolled in Part B when you become entitled to Part A unless you state that you don't want it. Although you do not have to purchase Part B, it is a good buy because the Federal government pays about 75 percent of the program costs. The Part B premium may be higher than $54 per month if you don't sign up for Part B when you first become eligible, unless you continue coverage in an employment-related health insurance plan after you become Medicare-eligible; the premium goes up 10 percent per year for each year you defer signing up.

Your Medicare card will show whether you have Hospital Insurance (Part A), Medical Insurance (Part B), or both, and the date your coverage started. If you have only one part of Medicare, you can get information about getting the other part from any Social Security office.

Medicare Hospital Insurance Benefits (Part A)

Medicare Part A helps pay for medically necessary inpatient care in a hospital, skilled nursing facility, or psychiatric hospital; for hospice care; for medically necessary home health care; and for wheelchairs, hospital beds, and other durable medical equipment supplied under the home health care benefit.

Medicare Part A hospital and skilled nursing facility benefits are paid on the basis of "benefit periods." A benefit period begins the first day you receive a Medicare-covered service in a qualified hospital. It ends when you have been out of a hospital or skilled nursing or rehabilitation facility for 60 days in a row. It also ends if you remain in a skilled nursing facility but do not receive any skilled care there for 60 days in a row.

If you enter a hospital again after 60 days, a new benefit period begins. With each new benefit period, all Part A hospital and skilled nursing facility benefits are renewed except for any "lifetime reserve days" or psychiatric hospital benefits that were used. There is no limit to the number of benefit periods you can have for hospital or skilled nursing facility care.

Inpatient Hospital Care

If you are hospitalized, as nearly 20 percent of Medicare beneficiaries are each year, Medicare will pay all charges for covered hospital services during the first 60 days of a benefit period except for the deductible. The Part A deductible in 2002 is $812 per benefit period. You are responsible for the deductible. In addition to the deductible, you are responsible for a share of the daily costs if your hospital stay lasts more than 60 days. For the 61st through the 90th day, Part A pays for all covered services except for coinsurance of $203 per day in 2002. You are responsible for the coinsurance.

Under Part A, you also have a lifetime reserve of 60 days for inpatient hospital care. These lifetime reserve days may be used whenever you are in the hospital for more than 90 consecutive days. When a reserve day is used, Part A pays for all covered services except for coinsurance of $406 in 2002. Again, the coinsurance is your responsibility. Once used, reserve days are not renewed.

Part A does not pay for—

- The first three pints of whole blood or units of packed cells used in each year. (To the extent the three-pint blood deductible is met under Part B, it does not have to be met under Part A.)
- A private hospital room, unless medically necessary, or a private duty nurse.
- Personal convenience items, such as a telephone or television in a hospital room.
- Care that is not medically necessary or for nonemergency care in a hospital not certified by Medicare.
- Care received outside the U.S. and its territories, except under limited circumstances in Canada and Mexico.

Skilled Nursing Facility Care

A skilled nursing facility (SNF) is a special kind of facility that primarily furnishes skilled nursing and rehabilitation services. It may be a separate facility or a distinct part of another facility, such as a hospital. Medicare benefits are payable only if you require daily skilled care that, as a practical matter, can only be provided in a skilled nursing facility on an inpatient basis, and the care is provided in a facility certified by Medicare. Medicare will not pay for your stay if the services you receive are primarily personal care or custodial services, such as assistance in walking, getting in and out of bed, eating, dressing, bathing, and taking medicine.

To qualify for Medicare coverage for skilled nursing facility care, you must have been in a hospital at least three consecutive days (not counting the day of discharge) before entering a skilled nursing facility. You must be admitted to the facility for the same condition for which you were treated in the hospital and the admission generally must be within 30 days of your discharge from the hospital. Your physician must certify that you need, and receive, skilled nursing or skilled rehabilitation services on a daily basis.

Medicare can help pay for up to 100 days of skilled care in a skilled nursing facility during a benefit period. All covered services for the first 20 days of care are fully paid by Medicare. All covered services for the next 80 days are paid by Medicare except for a daily coinsurance amount. The daily coinsurance amount in 2002 is $101.50. You are responsible for the coinsurance. If you require more than 100 days of care in a benefit period, you are responsible for all charges beginning with the 101st day.

Home Health Care

Medicare fully covers medically necessary home health visits if you are homebound, including part-time or intermittent skilled nursing services. A Medicare-certified home health agency can also furnish the services of physical and speech therapists. If you require speech-language pathology, physical therapy, continuing occupational therapy, or intermittent skilled nursing services, and if you are confined to your home and are under the care of a physician, Medicare can also pay for medical supplies, necessary part-time or intermittent home health aide services, occupational therapy, and medical social services. Coverage is also provided for a portion of the cost of wheelchairs, hospital beds, and other durable medical equipment provided under a plan-of-care set up and periodically reviewed by a physician. To qualify for Part A home health care coverage, you must have been released within the previous 14 days from a hospital where you stayed for at least three days or from a nursing home in which you were getting post-hospital care after a three-day or longer hospital stay.

Part A does not pay for—

- Full-time nursing care.
- Drugs.
- Meals delivered to your home.
- Twenty percent of the Medicare-approved amount for durable medical equipment, plus charges in excess of the approved amount on claims that are not "assigned" (see discussion of "accepting assignment," beginning on page 67).
- Homemaker services that are primarily to assist you in meeting personal care or housekeeping needs.

Hospice Care

Medicare beneficiaries certified as terminally ill may choose to receive hospice care rather than regular Medicare benefits for their terminal illness. If you enroll in a Medicare-certified hospice program, you will receive medical and support services necessary for symptom management and pain relief. When these services—which are most often provided in your home—are furnished by a Medicare-certified hospice program, the coverage includes physician services, nursing care, medical appliances and supplies (including drugs for symptom management and pain relief), short-term inpatient care, counseling, therapies, home health aide, and homemaker services.

You do not have to pay Medicare's deductibles and coinsurance for services and supplies furnished under the hospice benefit. You must pay only limited charges for outpatient drugs—up to $5 per prescription—and inpatient respite care (short-term care given to a hospice patient by another caregiver so that the usual caregiver can rest)—up to five percent of the Medicare-approved amount. In the event you require medical services for a condition unrelated to the terminal illness, regular Medicare benefits are available. When regular benefits are used, you are responsible for the applicable Medicare deductible and coinsurance amounts.

Psychiatric Hospital Care

Part A helps pay for up to 190 days of inpatient care in a Medicare-participating psychiatric hospital in your lifetime. Once you have used 190 days (or have used fewer than 190 days but have exhausted your inpatient hospital coverage), Part A doesn't pay for any more inpatient care in a psychiatric hospital. However, psychiatric care in general hospitals, rather than in freestanding psychiatric hospitals, is not subject to this 190-day limit. Inpatient psychiatric care in a general hospital is treated the same as other Medicare inpatient hospital care. If you are a patient in a psychiatric hospital on the first day of your entitlement to Medicare, there are additional limitations on the number of hospital days that Medicare will pay for.

Medicare Medical Insurance Benefits (Part B)

Part B helps pay for medically necessary physician services no matter where you receive them—at home, in the doctor's office, in a clinic, in a nursing home, or in a hospital. It also covers related medical services and supplies, medically necessary outpatient hospital services, X-rays, and laboratory tests. Coverage is also provided for certain ambulance services and the use at home of durable medical equipment, such as wheelchairs and hospital beds.

In addition, Part B covers you for medically necessary physical therapy, occupational therapy, and speech-language pathology services in a doctor's office, as an outpatient, or in your home. Various preventive and screening services are covered, including mammograms, Pap smears, colorectal cancer screening, diabetes monitoring, bone mass measurements, and flu, pneumococcal, and hepatitis B shots. Mental health services are covered. And if you qualify for home health care but do not have Part A, then Part B pays for all covered home health visits.

Outpatient prescription drugs generally are not covered by Part B. The exceptions include certain drugs furnished to hospice enrollees, non-self-administrable drugs provided as part of a physician's services, and special drugs, such as drugs furnished during the first year after an organ transplantation, crythropoctin for home dialysis patients, and certain oral cancer drugs.

When you use your Part B benefits, you will be required to pay the first $100 (the annual deductible) each calendar year before Medicare begins to pay for most covered services. The deductible must represent charges for services and supplies covered by Medicare. It also must be based on Medicare-approved amounts, not the actual charges billed by your physician or medical supplier.

After you meet the deductible, Part B generally pays 80 percent of the Medicare-approved amount for covered services you receive the rest of the year. You are responsible for the other 20 percent. But the rules vary depending on the service. For example, if you require home health services, you do not have to pay a deductible or coinsurance for the services, and you pay nothing for clinical laboratory services; on the other hand, you have to pay 50 percent of the approved amount for outpatient mental health services. The table on the next page summarizes Part B benefits.

You may also have other out-of-pocket costs under Part B if your physician or medical supplier does not accept "assignment" of your Medicare claim and charges more than Medicare's approved amount. The amount in excess of the approved amount is called the "excess charge" or "balance billing" and you are responsible for paying it. You should be aware, however, that there are certain charge limitations mandated by Federal law.

Medicare-Approved Amount

The Medicare-approved amount for physician services covered by Part B is based on a national fee schedule. The schedule assigns a dollar value to each physician service based on work, practice costs, and malpractice insurance costs. Under this payment system, each time you go to a physician for a service covered by Medicare, the amount Medicare will recognize for that service will be taken from the national fee schedule. Medicare generally pays 80 percent of that amount.

Because you can't tell in advance whether the approved amount and the actual charge for covered services and supplies will be the same, always ask your physicians and medical suppliers whether they accept "assignment" of Medicare claims.

Accepting Assignment

Those who take "assignment" on a Medicare claim agree to accept the Medicare-approved amount as payment in full. They are paid directly by Medicare, except for the deductible and coinsurance amounts that you must pay.

For example, for your first annual visit, if your physician accepts assignment, and the Medicare-approved amount for the service you receive is $200, you will be billed $120: $100 for the annual deductible plus 20 percent of the remaining $100, or $20. Medicare will pay the other $80. Having met the deductible for the year, the next time you use Part B services furnished by a physician or medical supplier who accepts assignment, you will be responsible for only 20 percent of the Medicare-approved amount.

Physicians and suppliers who sign Medicare "participation" agreements accept assignment on all Medicare claims. Their names and addresses are listed in the "Medicare Participating Physician/Supplier Directory," which is distributed to senior citizen organizations and should be available in all Social Security and Railroad Retirement Board offices, hospitals, and all state and area offices of the Administration on Aging. You can find a Medicare participating physician directory online at *www.medicare.gov*.

Even if your physician or supplier does not participate in Medicare, ask before receiving any services or supplies whether he or she will accept assignment of your Medicare claim. Many physicians and suppliers accept assignment on a case-by-case basis. If your physician or supplier will not accept assignment, you are responsible for paying all permissible charges. Medicare will then reimburse you its share of the approved amount for the services or supplies you received. Regardless of whether your physicians or other providers accept assignment, they are required to file your Medicare claim for you.

In certain situations, nonparticipating providers of services are required by law to accept assignment. For instance, all physicians and qualified laboratories must accept assignment for Medicare-covered clinical diagnostic laboratory tests. Physicians also must accept assignment

Summary of Part B Benefits

Part B Covers:	What you pay in 2002 if you have no supplemental (Medigap) coverage
Medical and other services: Doctor's services (except for routine physical exams), outpatient medical and surgical services and supplies, diagnostic tests, ambulatory surgery center facility fees for approved procedures, and durable medical equipment (such as wheelchairs, hospital beds, oxygen, and walkers). Also covers second surgical opinions, outpatient physical and occupational therapy including speech-language therapy, and outpatient mental health care.	**You pay:** • $100 deductible (pay once per calendar year). • 20 percent of approved amount after the deductible, except in the outpatient setting. • 20 percent for all outpatient physical, speech, and occupational therapy services. • 50 percent for most outpatient mental health.
Clinical laboratory services: Blood tests, urinalysis, and more.	**You pay:** • Nothing for services.
Home health care (with some limitations): Part-time skilled care, home health aide services, durable medical equipment when supplied by a home health agency while getting Medicare-covered home health care, and other supplies and services.	**You pay:** • Nothing for services. • 20 percent of approved amount for durable medical equipment.
Outpatient hospital services: Services for the diagnosis or treatment of an illness or an injury.	**You pay:** • A set copayment amount that varies according to the service.
Blood: Pints of blood needed as an outpatient, or as part of a Part B covered service.	**You pay:** • For the first three pints of blood, then 20 percent of the approved amount for additional pints of blood (after the deductible).
Preventive services: • Bone mass measurements for certain people with Medicare who are at risk for losing bone mass. • Colorectal cancer screening for all people with Medicare age 50 and older. Includes fecal occult blood test once every year*; flexible sigmoidoscopy once every four years; colonoscopy once every two years if you are high risk for cancer of the colon (no age limit); barium enema sigmoidoscopy or colonoscopy. • Diabetes monitoring including glucose monitors, test strips, lancets, and self-management training. • Mammogram screening for all women age 40 and older once every year. • Pap smear* and pelvic examination for all women with a clinical breast exam once every three years (once every year if you are high risk for cervical or vaginal cancer, or if you are of childbearing age and have had an abnormal Pap smear in the preceding three years. • Prostate cancer screening for all men age 50 and older. Includes digital rectal examination and Prostate Specific Antigen (PSA) test once every year.* • Vaccinations for all people. Includes flu shot once every year*; pneumonia shot (one may be all you ever need, ask your doctor)*; Hepatitis B shot (if you are at medium to high risk for hepatitis). *No deductible or coinsurance required.	**You pay:** • 20 percent of the Medicare-approved amount after the yearly Part B deductible except as noted.

Part B also helps pay for:
- Ambulance services (limited coverage).
- Artificial limbs and eyes.
- Braces—arm, leg, back, and neck.
- Chiropractic services (limited).
- Emergency care.
- Eyeglasses—one pair after cataract surgery with an intraocular lens.
- Kidney dialysis and kidney transplants.
- Medical supplies—items such as ostomy bags, surgical dressings, splints, casts, and some diabetic supplies.
- Outpatient prescription drugs (very limited).
- Prosthetic devices after mastectomy.
- Services of practitioners such as clinical psychologists, social workers, and nurse practitioners.
- Transplants—heart, lung, and liver (under certain conditions).
- X-rays and some other diagnostic tests.

for covered services provided to beneficiaries with incomes low enough to qualify for payment of their Medicare cost-sharing requirements through the Medicaid program.

Physician Charge Limits If a Physician Does Not Accept Assignment

While physicians who do not accept assignment of a Medicare claim can charge more than physicians who do, there is a limit on the amount they can charge you for services covered by Medicare. Under law, they are not permitted to charge more than 115 percent of the Medicare-approved amount for the service. Physicians who knowingly, willfully, and repeatedly charge more than the legal limit are subject to sanctions. If you think you have been overcharged, or you want to know what the limiting charge is for a particular service, contact the Medicare "carrier" for your area. You can find the name of the carrier by calling 1-800-633-4227 or checking *www.medicare.gov*. Limiting charge information also appears on the "Explanation of Medicare Benefits" form that you generally receive from the Medicare carrier when you go to a physician for a Medicare-covered service. You do not have to pay charges that exceed the legal limit.

If you think your physician has exceeded the charge limit, you should contact the physician and ask for a reduction in the charge, or a refund if you have paid more than the charge limit. If you cannot resolve the issue with the physician, you can call your Medicare carrier and ask for assistance.

More Charge Limits

Another Federal law requires physicians who do not accept assignment for elective surgery to give you a written estimate of your costs before the surgery if the total charge will be $500 or more. If the physician did not give you a written estimate, you are entitled to a refund of any amount you paid in excess of the Medicare-approved amount. Any nonparticipating physician who provides you with services that he or she knows or has reason to believe Medicare will determine to be medically unnecessary and thus will not pay for is required to so notify you in writing before performing the service. If written notice is not given, and you did not know that Medicare would not pay, you cannot be held liable to pay for that service. However, if you did receive written notice and signed an agreement to pay for the service, you will be held liable to pay.

More Doctors Taking Assignment

Until the last few years, "balance-billing" was a big problem for consumers. Many physicians did not take assignment and patients were left to pay a substantial portion of doctors' bills, since the bills were often substantially higher than the Medicare-approved payment. But balance-billing is less of a problem today. Because the difference between the Medicare-approved fee and what the physician can bill you is now limited to 15 percent, the amounts at stake are smaller than they once were. Also, more and more physicians are accepting assignment because the financial benefit to them of balance-billing is small. Under a special provision designed to encourage providers to take assignment, Medicare pays nonparticipating doctors only 95 percent of the Medicare fee schedule. Since the doctors can only balance-bill you for an amount equal to 15 percent of the Medicare-approved fee, the net effect is that the most a doctor can gain by balance-billing is less than 10 percent above what he or she would get by accepting assignment. The result has been that today more than 90 percent of approved charges are taken on assignment.

Other Gaps in Medicare Coverage for Doctors and Medical Suppliers (Part B)

In addition to the $100 annual deductible, your requirement to pay 20 percent coinsurance, and legally permissible charges in excess of the Medicare-approved amount for unassigned claims, there are other items that Medicare doesn't pay for—

- 50 percent of approved charges for most outpatient mental health treatment.
- Most services that are not reasonable and necessary for the diagnosis or treatment of an illness or injury.
- Most self-administrable prescription drugs or immunizations, except for pneumococcal, influenza, and hepatitis B vaccinations.
- Routine physicals and other screening services—except for mammograms, Pap smears, colorectal screening, diabetes monitoring, prostate cancer screening, glaucoma screening, and bone mass measurements at Medicare-approved intervals for beneficiaries who fall into categories Medicare has defined as eligible for these services.
- Dental care or dentures.
- Acupuncture treatment.
- Hearing aids or routine hearing loss examinations.
- Care received outside the United States and its territories, except under limited circumstances in Canada and Mexico.
- Routine foot care except when a medical condition affecting the lower limbs (such as diabetes) requires care by a medical professional.
- Services of naturopaths, Christian Science practitioners, or immediate relatives, or charges imposed by members of your household.
- The first three pints of whole blood or units of packed cells used in each year in connection with covered services. (To the extent the three-pint blood deductible is met under Part A, it does not have to be met under Part B.)
- Routine eye examinations or eyeglasses, except prosthetic lenses, if needed, after cataract surgery.

Types of Private Health Insurance

Several types of private health insurance arrangements are available to help consumers pay for services not covered by Medicare. You need to determine which type or types are available to you and meet your needs. We will discuss a number of options in the sections that follow. We do not recommend, and will not discuss here, the following two other options—

- Hospital indemnity plans, which pay specified cash amounts for inpatient hospital services. It is difficult for you to be sure that these amounts have kept up with current hospital charges or that they fit with Medicare benefits.
- Specified disease policies, which pay only when you need treatment for the insured disease. You can't anticipate the diseases that you might experience.

Another type of policy—a nursing home or long-term care policy—might make sense for you but is beyond the scope of this article.

Medigap Policies

Medigap insurance is regulated by Federal and state law and must be clearly identified as Medicare supplemental insurance. Unlike other types of health insurance, it is designed specifically to supplement Medicare's benefits by filling in some of the gaps in Medicare coverage.

To make it easier for consumers to comparison shop for Medigap insurance, nearly all states have adopted regulations that limit the number of different Medigap policies that can be sold to no more than 10 standard benefit plans, which have letter designations ranging from "A" through "J." See pages 74 and 75 for descriptions and comparisons of the 10 plans. Medigap insurers are also allowed to offer a high-deductible ($1,500) version of plans F and J.

Plan A of the 10 standard Medigap plans is the "basic" benefit package. Each of the other nine plans (B through J) includes the basic package plus a different combination of additional benefits. The plans cover specific expenses either not covered or not fully covered by Medicare. Insurers are not permitted to change the combination of benefits in any of the plans or to change the letter designations.

Each state must allow the sale of Plan A, and all Medigap insurers must make Plan A available. Insurers are not required to offer any of the other nine plans, but most offer several plans, and some offer all 10. Insurers can independently decide which of the nine optional plans they will sell as long as the plans they select have been approved for sale in the state in which they are to be offered.

To make it easier for consumers to compare plans and premiums, the same format, language, and definitions must be used in describing the benefits of each of the plans. A uniform chart and outline of coverage also must be used by the insurer to summarize those benefits for you.

As you shop for a Medigap policy, keep in mind that, for the same policy type, all companies coverages are alike, so they are competing on price, service, and reliability. Compare premiums and be satisfied that the insurer is reputable before buying.

Medigap policies pay most, if not all, Medicare coinsurance amounts and may provide coverage for Medicare's deductibles. Some of the 10 standard plans pay for services not covered by Medicare and some pay for charges in excess of Medicare's approved amount. Three cover half the cost of prescription drugs after a $250 deductible and up to $1,250 per year or $3,000 per year, depending on the plan. Look for the plan that best meets your needs. The plan features are summarized on page 74 and in the table on page 75.

Unlike some types of health coverage that restrict where and from whom you can receive care, Medigap policies are "fee-for-service" plans; they generally pay the same supplemental benefits regardless of your choice of health care provider. If Medicare pays for a service, wherever provided, the standard Medigap policy must pay its regular share of benefits. The only exception is Medicare SELECT insurance, discussed below.

How Your Health Condition and the Timing of Your Sign-up Affect the Medigap Coverage You Can Get

Medigap insurers are allowed to limit your coverage for "preexisting conditions." Preexisting conditions are generally health problems you went to see a physician about within the six months before the policy went into effect. Don't be misled by the phrase "no medical examination required"; you may still be required to report any preexisting conditions. If you have had a health problem, the insurer might not cover you immediately for expenses connected with that problem. Medigap policies, however, are required to cover preexisting conditions after the policy has been in effect for six months. Also, if you switch into a Medigap plan from another plan, the new plan can't impose a preexisting conditions waiting period for benefits covered under the previous plan beyond a six-month period counting from the time the benefits were first covered under the previous plan.

Preexisting exclusion provisions are not the only concern. Medigap insurers can also refuse to issue you a policy altogether if they are concerned about possible health conditions. But there are several important limits on their right to refuse you. The broadest guarantee you have of being able to get a Medigap policy is a provision requiring all Medigap insurers in your state to accept you into any of the plan types they offer if you are 65 or older and sign up within a period of six months from the date you first enrolled in Medicare Part B.

Many individuals are enrolled automatically in Part B as soon as they turn 65, or they sign up during an initial seven-month enrollment period that begins three months before they turn 65. If you are in this group, your Part B coverage generally starts in the month you turn 65 or shortly thereafter, depending on when you applied for Part B.

Others may delay their enrollment in Part B. For example, if after turning 65, you continue to work and choose to be continuously covered by an employer insurance plan, or if you are continuously covered under a spouse's employment-related insurance instead of Medicare Part B, you will have a special seven-month enrollment period for Part B. It begins with the month your or your spouse's work ends or when you are no longer covered under the employer plan, whichever comes first. Your six-month Medigap open enrollment period starts when your Part B coverage begins.

If you are covered under an employer group health plan when you become eligible for Part B at age 65, carefully consider your options. Once you enroll in Part B, the six-month Medigap open enrollment period starts and cannot be extended or repeated.

If you are 65 or older and are eligible for Part B and never signed up for it, you may buy Part B during Medicare's annual general enrollment period. It runs from January 1 through March 31. If you sign up during the annual Part B enrollment period, both your Part B coverage and Medigap open enrollment period begin the following July 1.

Your Medicare card shows the effective dates for your Part A and/or Part B coverage. To figure whether you are in your Medigap open enrollment period, add six months to the effective date of your Part B coverage. If the date is in the future and you are at least 65, you are eligible for open enrollment. If the date is in the past, you are not eligible.

There are certain other circumstances in which Medigap insurers are required to accept you:

- All Medigap insurers are required by law to accept you into any of the plan types they offer if you enrolled in a managed care plan, Medicare private fee-for-service plan, or Medical Savings Account plan when you first became eligible at age 65 and disenrolled from that plan within one year.
- All Medigap insurers are required by law to accept you in any of plan types A, B, C, or F that they offer if—
  - ➡ Your employer terminated a Medicare supplemental plan that covered you.
  - ➡ You lost coverage under a managed care plan, Medicare private fee-for-service plan, or Medical Savings Account plan because the plan was terminated, you moved out of the plan's service area, or you disenrolled because the plan failed to meet contract provisions.
  - ➡ Your previous Medigap insurer became insolvent, violated coverage provisions, or misrepresented its policy's provisions.
- Your previous Medigap insurer is required to take you back into a policy of the same coverage type you last had with it if (1) you left it to enroll in a managed care plan, Medicare private fee-for-service plan, Medical Savings Account plan, or Medicare SELECT plan; (2) you had not previously been enrolled in such a plan; and (3) you then disenrolled from the new plan within one year.

If a Medigap insurer is required to insure you under these rules, the insurer can't deny or condition the issuance or effectiveness, or discriminate in the pricing, of a policy because of your medical history, health status, or claims experience. The company can, however, impose the same preexisting conditions restrictions that it applies to other Medigap policies, and you will have to enroll in the Medigap plan within 63 days of the time your other coverage terminates.

Although Medigap companies are not required to accept you unless you fall into the categories we've described, in many parts of the country at least a few companies offer "guaranteed-issue" policies. These policies are available to any consumer, regardless of health condition. They may impose preexisting conditions limits, however.

Among companies that are not guaranteed-issue, some turn down applicants for very minor medical problems, but others are more flexible. Try several companies. The fact that one turns you down doesn't mean another won't accept you.

Once you have been accepted for a Medigap policy, the company is required by law to renew your policy unless you choose to cancel or stop paying premiums. Although Medigap insurers must renew their policies, they can raise their premiums—so long as they treat all policyholders similarly—and higher premiums could make a policy unattractive or unaffordable for you.

Keep in mind that the rights to enroll and renew and the limits on pre-existing conditions exclusions we've discussed here apply only to Medigap policies issued after Federal requirements went into effect in 1992 (Plans A through J). A policy you get through your employer or that you signed up for before age 65 or before 1992 might not have these protections.

Older Medigap Policies

Current Federal requirements generally do not apply to Medigap policies in force before 1992. You don't have to switch to one of the 10 standard plans if you have an older policy that is guaranteed renewable. But you may want to consider switching to a standardized Medigap plan if its premiums, benefits, or services are superior and the insurer is willing to accept you.

If you do switch, you will not be allowed to go back to the old policy. Before switching, compare benefits and premiums, and determine if there are waiting periods for any of the benefits in the new policy. Some of the older policies may provide superior coverage, especially for prescription drugs and extended skilled nursing care.

If you had the old Medigap policy at least six months and you decide to switch, the new policy is not permitted to impose a waiting period for a preexisting condition if you satisfied a waiting period for a similar benefit under your old policy. If, however, a benefit is included in the new policy that was not in the old policy, a waiting period of up to six months may be applied to that particular benefit.

An important point: if you have a pre-1992 policy, it might not include a guaranteed right to renew. By switching to a Medigap policy—if you can get one—you get that right for the future.

Medicare SELECT

You may want to consider a Medicare SELECT policy. Medicare SELECT policies, which may be offered by insurance companies and HMOs, are the same as standard Medigap insurance in nearly all respects. If you buy a Medicare SELECT policy, you are buying one of the 10 standard Medigap plans.

The only difference between Medicare SELECT and standard Medigap insurance is that Medicare SELECT policies will pay or provide full supplemental benefits only if covered services are obtained through specified health care professionals and facilities. Medicare SELECT policies can be expected to have lower premiums because of this limitation. The specified health care professionals and facilities, called "preferred providers," are selected by the insurance company or HMO. Each issuer of a Medicare SELECT policy makes arrangements with its own network of preferred providers.

If you have a Medicare SELECT policy, each time you receive covered services from a preferred provider, Medicare will pay its share of the approved charges and the insurer will pay or provide the full supplemental benefits provided for in the policy. Medicare SELECT insurers also must pay supplemental benefits for emergency health care furnished by providers outside the preferred provider network. In general, Medicare SELECT policies deny payment or pay less than the full benefit if you go outside the network for nonemergency services. Medicare, however, will still pay its share of approved charges if the services you receive outside the network are services covered by Medicare.

Managed Care Plans That Contract with Medicare

An alternative to purchasing a Medigap policy is enrolling in a managed care plan that participates in what Medicare calls the "Medicare + Choice" program. The managed care plan might be—

- An HMO;
- A provider-sponsored organization (PSO), which is much like an HMO except that it is organized around an affiliation of a hospital or hospitals and a group of doctors and other providers; or
- A preferred provider organization (PPO).

Of these three types, currently only HMOs are available in most parts of the country, but the others might become more broadly available in the future.

About 15 percent of all Medicare beneficiaries have enrolled in managed care plans. As of 2002, about 60 percent of beneficiaries had access to at least one Medicare managed care plan serving their geographic area.

Medicare makes a monthly payment to each managed care plan to cover Medicare's share of the cost of the services you receive. While you are in one of these plans, you have no Medicare coverage other than coverage through the plan; if the plan doesn't cover a service or expense, you are on your own.

Many Medicare HMO plans charge enrollees a monthly premium, but as of 2002, about 30 percent of beneficiaries had access to a plan that charged no premium. (You do still have to pay your Medicare Part B premium.) Most plans require enrollees to share in the costs of covered services by paying deductibles, coinsurance, or copayments (for instance, $10 per office visit) as services are used. Studies indicate that this cost-sharing costs enrollees an average of about $27 per month in addition to any premium charges. Plans that don't charge premiums tend to have higher cost-sharing requirements.

A managed care plan must arrange to provide you all Part A and Part B services (if you are covered by both parts of Medicare). And the cost to you of these plans' copayments or other charges for these services must not exceed the cost of the copayments and deductibles for these services under traditional Medicare.

Medicare HMO plans provide some types of coverage that you might otherwise have to pay for out-of-pocket (or through a Medigap plan). For example, many of these HMOs provide coverage for prescription drugs, extra hospital days, routine physical exams, and hearing aids.

You can find out which, if any, Medicare managed care plans are available to you by calling Medicare at 1-800-633-4227 or by using the Medicare Health Plan Compare feature at *www.medicare.gov*. You can get details on the plans from the plans themselves or from Medicare Health Plan Compare.

Enrollment in a Medicare HMO can be a very good deal for many consumers. For zero premium or a relatively small premium in most HMOs, you can get coverage at least as full as you'd get with the Medigap "F" plan, which costs most policyholders a premium of more than $1,200 per year. For a couple, that means you might save more than $2,400 per year by being in an HMO.

If you enroll in an HMO, you will generally be covered *only for services you receive through the HMO's network of providers and only for services given by your primary care doctor or given based on a referral by your primary care doctor*. There are limited exceptions to these rules—

- Plans must pay for emergency services from non-participating providers if you get care in what a "prudent" person with an average knowledge of medical care would reasonably believe to be an emergency. The care is covered until the treating physician determines that you are stabilized for discharge or transfer.
- Plans must pay for non-emergency "urgent" care if you need out-of-area care for an unforeseen illness, injury, or condition and it is not feasible to get services from the plan, if you travel outside the plan's service area and need kidney dialysis, or if you need post-stabilization care after an out-of-area emergency.
- Plans can't require a primary care doctor's referral for a woman who wants to go directly to a network doctor for routine or preventive women's health care services.
- Plans must have procedures to identify enrollees with complex or grave medical conditions and to set up treatment plans for these enrollees with an appropriate number of covered visits to specialists without the need for a referral before each visit.

Some HMO plans may offer a "point of service" (POS) provision. With a POS HMO plan, you will be able to go to providers outside the plan's network, or to in-network providers without a referral, and still have the plan pay a portion of the bill. But if you go out of network, you will probably have higher out-of-pocket costs than if you stay within the plan. You will probably have to pay deductibles and coinsurance amounts—say, 20 percent of the non-network provider's bill. But even if you go out of network in a POS plan, the plan will be required to put a cap on out-of-pocket costs, and non-network providers will not be allowed to bill for more than the fee that would be allowed under the traditional Medicare program.

PPO plans give members even more flexibility than a POS HMO plan. In a PPO, you are able to self-refer for any covered service. You are able to use any provider of your choice, but if you use a non-network provider, you can expect to pay a higher deductible amount and higher coinsurance amounts than if you stay within the plan's provider network. As of this writing, Medicare managed care PPO plans are available only in parts of Pennsylvania and Ohio.

You are eligible to enroll in a Medicare managed care plan if you live in the plan's service area, are enrolled in Medicare Part B, do not have permanent kidney failure, and have not elected the Medicare hospice benefit. The plan must enroll Medicare beneficiaries in the order of application, without health screening, during at least one open enrollment period each year.

A big advantage of these Medicare managed care plans for many Medicare recipients is that the plans must accept you regardless of your medical condition. If you can't qualify for a Medigap policy because of a health problem, you can join a Medicare managed care plan.

Unfortunately, many HMOs available to consumers and businesses have not chosen to contract with Medicare, and some that have include only a portion of their entire service area under the contract.

Even the fact that Medicare HMOs restrict coverage to care authorized and delivered by their participating providers may not be as significant a limitation as it seems. If you join a Medicare-contracting HMO and you're not satisfied with the care you're receiving, you can quit. In the year 2002, you might be locked in for as much as six months, and starting in 2003, you might be locked in for a year, but you are never locked in permanently. By quitting, you resume your full regular fee-for-service Medicare coverage, and you can enroll in a traditional Medigap plan or you can try another HMO. If you quit and want to join a Medigap plan, of course, the Medigap plan might choose not to accept you if you have a medical problem (subject to the special rules on Medigap enrollment discussed above). But in most areas there is at least one Medigap plan that is "guaranteed issue"—meaning you can't be turned down. What's more, no Medicare HMO is permitted to turn you down.

This flexibility is reassuring, but you still will want to study your options carefully before joining a Medicare-contracting HMO. Be sure to read the plan's membership materials carefully to learn your rights and the nature and extent of your coverage. Compare benefits, costs, provider choices, and other features to determine which plan best meets your needs.

Employer Group Insurance

For Retirees

About a third of all Medicare beneficiaries have insurance to supplement their basic Medicare coverage through the companies where they were employed prior to retirement. If you or your spouse is an active employee with employer-sponsored coverage, find out if coverage can be continued when you retire. Check the price and the benefits for you and your spouse.

Group health insurance that is continued after retirement usually has the advantage of having no waiting periods or exclusions for preexisting conditions, and the coverage is usually based on group premium rates, which may be lower than the premium rates for individually purchased policies.

But if a spouse under 65 was covered under the employer policy, make sure you know what effect continued coverage of the over-65 retired spouse will have on the under-65 retired spouse's insurance protection. Also, since employer group insurance policies do not have to comply with the Federal minimum benefit standards for Medigap policies, it is important to determine what coverage your specific retirement policy provides. The policy might not provide the same benefits as a Medigap policy. On the other hand, it might offer other benefits such as prescription drug coverage and routine dental care.

For Working Persons Age 65 or Over

If you are 65 or over, you or your spouse works, and you have coverage through an employer group plan, that plan will be the primary payer of claims and Medicare will be secondary. This means that the employer plan pays first on your hospital and medical bills. If the employer plan does not pay all of your expenses, Medicare pays secondary benefits for Medicare-covered services to supplement the amount paid by the employer plan.

Employers who have 20 or more employees are required to offer the same health benefits, under the same conditions, to employees age 65 or over and to employees' spouses who are 65 or over, that they offer to younger employees and spouses. Employers with fewer than 20 employees may or may not choose to offer health insurance to employees age 65 and over.

You may accept or reject coverage under an employer group health plan. If you accept the employer plan, it will be your primary payer. If you reject the plan, Medicare will be the primary payer for Medicare-covered health services that you receive. If you reject the employer plan, you can buy supplemental insurance but an employer cannot provide you with a plan that pays supplemental benefits for Medicare-covered services or subsidize such coverage. An employer may, however, offer a plan that pays for health care services not covered by Medicare, such as hearing aids, routine dental care, and physical checkups.

A New Type of Coverage

A new type of coverage was authorized by 1997 Federal legislation: private fee-for-service plans. In a plan of this type, Medicare makes a premium payment on your behalf to a private insurance company, you pay any additional premium the company requires, and you get whatever package of benefits the company offers (not less than the coverage you would get under traditional Medicare). During the time you are enrolled in a Medicare private fee-for-service plan, Medicare will make no payments for services you receive. Providers, including doctors, hospitals, and home health agencies, that contract with the plan are allowed to balance-bill you (make you pay out of your own pocket) up to 15 percent above the plan's payment rate for services provided. Depending on how a private fee-for-service plan structures itself, it can function, from the consumer's standpoint, much like basic Medicare combined with a Medigap plan.

As of this writing, private fee-for-service plan options were available only in certain regions of the country. The most widely available option, Sterling Option I, had a premium in Illinois, for example, of $78 per month (in addition to the $54 Medicare Part B premium). That is comparable to premiums in some Medigap plans. The plan's benefit structure included paying: the full cost of unlimited hospital days after a $350 per stay deductible, the full cost of 100 skilled nursing home days after a $25 per day copayment, 65 percent of the cost of home health care visits, and the cost of doctor visits after a $20 per visit copayment. You can check on current availability and premiums and benefits of private fee-for-service plans by calling Medicare at 1-800-633-4227 or using the Medicare Health Plan Compare feature at *www.medicare.gov*.

The rules for disenrolling from private fee-for-service plans are the same as the rules for disenrolling from Medicare HMOs.

Shopping for Coverage

You must decide what type of plan you want— whether you want coverage through an employer plan (if one is available to you), through a Medigap policy, through an HMO that has a contract with Medicare, or through a private fee-for-service plan. Once you decide on a type of plan, you will have to decide which specific benefit package you want and choose a specific company. Naturally, it is important to shop for the best deal.

In choosing a type of plan, you will want to consider many factors, including—

- The doctors and other providers who will be available to you. If you have providers you are happy with, will they be available through the plan?
- The control you will have over the care you get. Will your care be limited to what your primary care doctor will recommend? How likely is it that even care your doctor recommends will be denied by the plan?
- Your costs—both premiums and out-of-pocket costs (for deductibles and copayments and services and supplies not covered by the plan).
- The quality of care you can expect. Will you be able to find a plan that screens out low-quality providers, assists its providers in providing the highest quality care, and does not obstruct your access to needed care?
- Coverage when you are away from home. Will you be able to get care

when traveling or if you are regularly in another part of the country for extended periods of time?

Shopping for a Medigap Policy

If you decide to consider Medigap policies, you will have to decide which plan you want. You can use the plan descriptions on pages 74 and 75. Then compare premiums and other features offered by competing companies. You can get a listing of available companies in your area by calling Medicare at 1-800-633-4227 or using the Medicare Personal Plan Finder at *www.medicare.gov*. You'll want to check several points on each policy.

One of the most important and confusing questions is how premiums are set. There are three main possibilities. "Community-rated" policies have the same rates for all policyholders in the same geographic area, regardless of how old they are when they sign up. For example, if the premium is $1,000, it will be $1,000 for a 65-year-old and an 80-year-old whether they signed up 10 years ago or today. This is the simplest rate structure and the one most in keeping with the pure insurance concept of broadly shared risk.

"Issue-age-rated" policies set your premium based on your age when you buy the policy. The rate doesn't go up as a policyholder ages except to the extent that inflation, claims experience, or some other business reason causes the company to raise its prices across the board. If the rate for a 65-year-old just signing up is $900, it might be $1,100 for a 70-year-old just signing up, but the premium for someone who signs up at age 65 will remain $900 as he or she ages (except for across-the-board price increases). If two 70-year-olds have the same policy and one bought it at age 65 while the other bought it at age 70, the latter person's premiums will be higher. But under most companies' issue-age-rated plans, two persons who bought plans at the same age will pay the same premiums even if one is years older than the other.

"Attained-age-rated" policies charge escalating premiums for the same policyholder as the policyholder ages. If the rate for a 65-year-old just signing up is $800 and that policyholder holds the policy until age 75, the premium for him or her at age 75 might be $1,200. Most companies that offer attained-age-rated policies charge persons of the same age the same premium whether a person signed up today or signed up years earlier.

With community-rated policies, younger policyholders subsidize older policyholders, who tend to be sicker and more costly to insure. As a result, community-rated policies tend to be more attractive for older than for younger consumers. With an issue-age policy, you overpay for yourself when you are young in order to have relatively low rates as you grow older. As a result, policyholders with issue-age policies are not likely to benefit from switching policies after they've had a policy for five or 10 years. With attained-age policies, you pay at each age according to the insurance company's expected costs for someone of your age. Persons with attained-age policies will benefit by continuing every few years to compare pricing of other policies they qualify for and consider switching.

After you know the method used to set premiums, you will need to find out actual premiums for any companies you want to consider. Attained-age policies are the most difficult to shop for because you need to check not only the premium at your age of purchase but also the built-in premium increases based on age.

You have to be very careful comparing premiums between issue-age policies and attained-age policies. An attained-age policy that looks very inexpensive for a 65-year-old at the age of purchase might not look so good when premium increases based on age are taken into account. A comparison of premiums recently offered by two different companies for plan F in Maryland illustrates the point. Company A sells attained-age policies; Company B sells issue-age policies. Company A's premiums were $996 for a 65-year-old but were $1,809 for an 80-year-old; these

Standard Medigap Plans

Following is a list of the 10 standard plans and the benefits provided by each:

PLAN A (the basic policy) consists of these basic benefits:

- Coverage for the Part A coinsurance amount ($203 per day in 2002) for the 61st through the 90th day of hospitalization in each Medicare benefit period.
- Coverage for the Part A coinsurance amount ($406 per day in 2002) for each of Medicare's 60 nonrenewable lifetime hospital inpatient reserve days used.
- After all Medicare hospital benefits are exhausted, coverage for 100 percent of the Medicare Part A eligible hospital expenses. Coverage is limited to a maximum of 365 days of additional inpatient hospital care during the policyholder's lifetime. This benefit is paid either at the rate Medicare pays hospitals under its Prospective Payment System or another appropriate standard of payment.
- Coverage under Medicare Parts A and B for the reasonable cost of the first three pints of blood or equivalent quantities of packed red blood cells per calendar year unless replaced in accordance with federal regulations.
- Coverage for the coinsurance amount for Part B services (generally 20 percent of approved amount; 50 percent of approved charges for mental health services) after $100 annual deductible is met.

PLAN B includes the basic benefits *plus*:
- Coverage for the Medicare Part A inpatient hospital deductible ($812 per benefit period in 2002).

PLAN C includes the basic benefits *plus*:
- Coverage for the Medicare Part A deductible.
- Coverage for the skilled nursing facility care coinsurance amount ($101.50 per day for days 21 through 100 per benefit period in 2002).
- Coverage for the Medicare Part B deductible ($100 per calendar year in 2002).
- 80 percent coverage for medically necessary emergency care in a foreign country, after a $250 deductible.

PLAN D includes the basic benefits *plus*:
- Coverage for the Medicare Part A

deductible. Coverage for the skilled nursing facility care daily coinsurance amount.
- 80 percent coverage for medically necessary emergency care in a foreign country, after a $250 deductible.
- Coverage for at-home recovery. The at-home recovery benefit pays up to $1,600 per year for short-term, at-home assistance with activities of daily living (bathing, dressing, personal hygiene, etc.) for those recovering from an illness, injury, or surgery. There are various benefit requirements and limitations.

PLAN E includes the basic benefits *plus*:
- Coverage for the Medicare Part A deductible.
- Coverage for the skilled nursing facility care daily coinsurance amount.
- 80 percent coverage for medically necessary emergency care in a foreign country, after a $250 deductible.
- Coverage for preventive medical care. The preventive medical care benefit pays up to $120 per year for such things as a physical examination, flu shot, serum cholesterol screening, hearing test, diabetes screenings, and thyroid function test.

PLAN F includes the basic benefits *plus*:
- Coverage for the Medicare Part A deductible.
- Coverage for the skilled nursing facility care daily coinsurance amount.
- Coverage for the Medicare Part B deductible.
- 80 percent coverage for medically necessary emergency care in a foreign country, after a $250 deductible.
- Coverage for 100 percent of Medicare Part B excess charges.*

PLAN G includes the basic benefits *plus*:
- Coverage for the Medicare Part A deductible. Coverage for the skilled nursing facility care daily coinsurance amount.
- Coverage for 80 percent of Medicare Part B excess charges.*
- 80 percent coverage for medically necessary emergency care in a foreign country, after a $250 deductible.
- Coverage for at-home recovery (see Plan D).

PLAN H includes the basic benefits *plus*:
- Coverage for the Medicare Part A deductible. Coverage for the skilled nursing facility care daily coinsurance amount.
- 80 percent coverage for medically necessary emergency care in a foreign country, after a $250 deductible.
- Coverage for 50 percent of the cost of prescription drugs up to a maximum annual benefit of $1,250 after the policyholder meets a $250 per year deductible (this is called the "basic" prescription drug benefit).

PLAN I includes the basic benefits *plus*:
- Coverage for the Medicare Part A deductible. Coverage for the skilled nursing facility care daily coinsurance amount.
- Coverage for 100 percent of Medicare Part B excess charges.*
- Basic prescription drug coverage (see Plan H).
- 80 percent coverage for medically necessary emergency care in a foreign country, after a $250 deductible.
- Coverage for at-home recovery (see Plan D).

PLAN J includes the basic benefits *plus*:
- Coverage for the Medicare Part A deductible.
- Coverage for the skilled nursing facility care daily coinsurance amount.
- Coverage for the Medicare Part B deductible.
- Coverage for 100 percent of Medicare Part B excess charges.*
- 80 percent coverage for medically necessary emergency care in a foreign country, after a $250 deductible.
- Coverage for preventive medical care (see Plan E).
- Coverage for at-home recovery (see Plan D).
- Coverage for 50 percent of the cost of prescription drugs up to a maximum annual benefit of $3,000 after the policyholder meets a $250 per year deductible (this is called the "extended" prescription drug benefit).

* Plan pays a specified percentage of the difference between Medicare's approved amount for Part B services and the actual charges (up to the amount of charge limitations set by either Medicare or state law).

premiums applied regardless of how old the policyholder was when the policy was purchased. In contrast, Company B's premium for a policy-holder who purchased the policy at age 65 was $1,068 regardless of that person's current age. Company A's $996 premium for a 65-year-old beats the $1,068 Company B premium. But Company A's $1,809 premium for an 80-year-old is substantially higher than the $1,068 Company B figure.

In addition to checking on each policy's way of calculating premiums and its actual premiums, you'll want to consider—

- Is there a waiting period before preexisting conditions are covered? If so, how long is it?
- Is it a guaranteed-issue policy? In other words, can you sign up regardless of your medical condition?

In addition to checking cost, benefit, and service quality information, you might want to check how financially sound companies are. Even if a company goes out of business, you will probably be protected under state insurance provisions for claims you already have. But financial soundness is important for this reason: if your company were to go out of business when you had a medical condition that companies don't want to cover, you might have a hard time finding new coverage. You can ask an insurance company or an agent for the company's rating with A. M. Best, a service that rates financial soundness. A rating of "A+" or "A" is a good sign (but not a guarantee). You can also find financial soundness ratings on most plans by calling Weiss Research at 1-800-289-9222 or visiting *www.weissratings.com*. The Weiss fee per company is $15 by phone and $7.95 online.

Shopping for an HMO

In some respects, comparing HMOs is easier than comparing Medigap plans. You know that HMO coverage is guaranteed-issue (the HMO can't refuse to accept you), that there can be no preexisting condition limitations, and that paperwork will be simple. Also, the rates are simple. Most HMOs offer only one or two packages of benefits and premiums under their Medicare contracts. A plan's premiums apply to all ages and to all locations within the service area. But there are key respects in which comparing HMOs is more difficult than comparing Medigap policies.

One plan comparison challenge results from the fact that there are no standard benefit packages for Medicare HMOs. You will need to find out each HMO's special benefit features. Consider, for example—

- Prescription drug coverage
- Limits on hospital days

- Copayments required
- Eye exam and lens coverage
- Hearing exam and hearing aid coverage
- Dental care coverage
- Mental health service coverage
- Coverage for extended nursing home stays

The most important impact on a substantial number of beneficiaries is likely to result from differences in prescription drug coverage. For example, someone who has a moderate need for prescription drugs is likely to have $700 more in out-of-pocket prescription drug expenses in some plans than in others serving the same area.

An even more important and difficult issue when comparing Medicare HMOs is the possibility of quality differences. As we have noted elsewhere in this book, HMOs have much more control over the quality of care their enrollees receive than fee-for-service Medigap plans have. With an HMO, you are limited in your choice of providers and you are covered only for services your primary care provider authorizes. In addition, some HMOs take a proactive role in assuring that you get preventive care and that your care is coordinated and managed effectively.

The information on the Plan Ratings table in Chapter 4 will help you judge the quality of health care and service in many HMOs.

What Is Covered By Standard Medigap Plans

	Medigap Plans									
	A	B	C	D	E	F	G	H	I	J

All Medigap plans include coverage for your share of the costs of all Part A hospital inpatient days for up to 365 days, the costs of three pints of blood under parts A and B, and your 20 percent coinsurance share for Part B services.

Extra Benefits	A	B	C	D	E	F	G	H	I	J
Skilled nursing facility coinsurance (days 21-100)			✓	✓	✓	✓	✓	✓	✓	✓
Part A deductible		✓	✓	✓	✓	✓	✓	✓	✓	✓
Part B deductible			✓			✓				✓
Part B excess charges						100%	80%		100%	100%
Foreign travel emergency			✓	✓	✓	✓	✓	✓	✓	✓
At-home recovery				✓			✓		✓	✓
Prescription drugs								_1	_1	_2
Preventive medical care					✓					✓

Two prescription drug benefits are offered by Medigap plans:

[1] A "basic" benefit with a $250 annual deductible, 50 percent coinsurance, and a $1,250 maximum annual benefit (Plans H and I above); and

[2] An "extended" benefit (Plan J above) containing a $250 annual deductible, 50 percent coinsurance, and a $3,000 maximum annual benefit.

Chapter 7

Finding a Good Doctor

Whatever health plan you choose, the quality of care you receive will depend heavily on your primary care doctor.

Your primary care doctor should be a general practitioner, family practitioner, internist, or pediatrician (for children), or perhaps an obstetrician/gynecologist (for women). If you are in an HMO, you won't be allowed to get your primary care from any other specialty. But even if you have traditional insurance, you are better off not to rely on a more narrow specialist—say, a surgeon—for primary care because a specialist may see the cures for your health problems in the tasks he or she is skilled to perform—surgery, perhaps, where drug therapy would suffice.

A good relationship with a primary care physician is important for several reasons. First, the doctor is someone you can trust and talk openly with if a serious medical problem arises. Second, the doctor is familiar with your medical history, your family relationships, and other factors that can help in diagnosing the physical and emotional causes of health problems. Third, the doctor is there to guide and coordinate your care through the rest of the health care system—to refer you to specialists, for instance, or to meet you at the emergency department to oversee your care after an accident.

You might want to begin the search for a primary care doctor even before you select a health plan: find one or more good doctors, find out which plan or plans the doctors participate in, and choose one of those plans. But many consumers will wait to choose a doctor until after they have selected a health plan.

If you have selected an indemnity-type plan, you'll have a choice among all doctors in the community (except those who aren't accepting new patients). HMO members will have to choose doctors who participate in their plans, and PPO and point of service HMO members will probably want to choose participating doctors.

HMO and PPO members can start by checking their plan's provider list. Many of these lists include a few facts on each physician's credentials. You may be able to get additional information—or help narrowing your choices—by calling the plan's member services staff. Some of the most progressive plans actually list on their websites a few quality measures about their physicians, including the results of patient satisfaction surveys. You might check the websites of plans in your area—including plans of which you are not a member—to see if any have such useful information.

If you are a member of an indemnity plan or you have not yet chosen a plan, you have several ways to start your search. (You can also use these approaches if you are a member of a PPO or HMO, although they may lead you to some doctors who aren't good candidates because they don't participate in your plan.)

One approach is to use an independently researched, published list of recommended physicians. *Consumers' CHECKBOOK* publishes such a list, our *Guide to Top Doctors*, which lists the doctors most often recommended by other doctors in a survey in which 260,000 doctors in the 50 largest metropolitan areas in the U.S. were asked to name the one or two

doctors, in each of 35 specialties, whom they "would consider most desirable for care of a loved one." This *Guide* can be ordered for $19.95 from Checkbook's Doctor Guide, 733 15th Street, NW, Suite 820, Washington, DC 20005. Or you can subscribe for two years of online use of the *Guide* at *www.checkbook.org*. Other lists of good doctors are sometimes published by other independent groups in various parts of the country. Independence is important; there is little or no value in the many 800-number services and websites that are created by commercial entities that simply charge doctors to be listed or that are created by hospitals and medical groups to promote their affiliated physicians.

Another good approach for identifying candidates to be your doctor is to ask friends and associates for recommendations. Our studies have shown that consumers tend to identify and recommend doctors that other doctors also recommend.

Still another approach, if you have moved, is to ask a doctor you have known in some other part of the country for recommendations. If you have been forced to change doctors because you've changed plans and your doctor from the previous plan doesn't participate, ask that doctor to recommend a doctor from the provider list of the new plan.

You might also want to call a high-quality hospital for referrals. If you call a hospital, simply call the main switchboard and ask for someone who makes referrals to family doctors. Good sources of prospects are teaching hospitals, where you can ask specifically for doctors who have teaching responsibilities. Although the full-time faculty at the local medical schools may include only a handful of primary care physicians, a surprisingly large number of doctors teach—often putting in two or three hours per week in clinical work with medical students and interns while maintaining their own practices. The teaching experience exposes the doctor to new medical developments and to continuing challenges to his or her own standards of practice.

Part-time teaching doctors at hospitals affiliated with medical schools are excellent prospects, but so are doctors who teach at large community hospitals.

Two national directories can help you in your search: the *American Medical Directory* and the *Directory of Medical Specialists*. Both list a few key facts about physicians. They are available at most large libraries, and links to the Web versions of both sources can be found at *www.checkbook.org*.

When you have identified a few potential candidates, you will want to ask some questions about each. A few can be answered from published directories; others will require a call to the doctor's office; and still others can be answered only by checking with other patients or by meeting—or using—the doctor. The following are a few of the more important questions.

- *Does the doctor work as a personal, or family, doctor on a primary care basis? For children, adults, or both?*
- *Is the doctor taking new patients?*

- *How convenient is the doctor's office? Is there public transportation? Parking? Access for the handicapped?*
- *Is the doctor "board certified" in his or her specialty?* Although a well-recommended doctor who is not "board certified" may serve you admirably, there seems to be little reason not to seek out certification, which means that the doctor has taken at least two to six years of post-medical school training and has passed a difficult exam.
- *Where did the doctor take his or her residency?* If the hospital where the doctor took advanced post-medical school training—called a "residency"—has a recognizable university tie, this almost assures that the doctor received good instruction—for instance, Stanford University Hospital or Johns Hopkins Hospital. But just because you can't recognize a university connection in the name of the hospital does not mean there is none. Harvard University uses Massachusetts General, for example.
- *What medical school did the doctor attend?* Virtually all medical schools in the United States are acknowledged to be of relatively high quality. A few other countries, such as Canada, Britain, Switzerland, and Belgium, have schools of comparable quality. So give special consideration to doctors who went to school in one of these countries. But remember that most experts think the location of a physician's residency is more revealing than the medical school attended.
- *When did the doctor graduate from medical school?* This tells you roughly how old the doctor is and how fresh his or her training is. You may prefer a doctor who has years of practical experience, who has seen firsthand a vast range of medical problems. But unless this doctor is actively involved in teaching or continuing education programs, he or she may not be aware of many recent medical care developments.
- *At what hospitals can the doctor admit patients?* You do well to have a doctor who can admit patients both at a major teaching hospital and at a good community hospital. You'll want the doctor to be able to consider sending you to the teaching hospital if you have a complex or high-risk medical problem but to be able to send you to a good community hospital—which is likely to be more pleasant—if your case is simple. To identify good hospitals, you might consult another *Consumers' CHECKBOOK* resource, published in hard copy and on the Web: *Consumers' Guide to Hospitals.* This *Guide* rates hospitals based on death rates and rates of complications, ratings by physicians, scores given by accreditation reviewers, and other measures. This *Guide* can be ordered for $19.95 from Checkbook's Hospital Guide, 733 15th Street, NW, Suite 820, Washington, DC 20005. Or you can subscribe for two years of online use of the *Guide* at *www.checkbook.org.*
- *Does the doctor have teaching responsibilities at a hospital?* If you found the doctor's name through a hospital referral service, you may already have this answer. The answer is important because a teaching position reflects respect from colleagues and also assures that the doctor is regularly exposed to new developments and to questions from medical students and residents.
- *Does the doctor practice in a group or alone?* Doctors who share an office may share ideas and maintain informal standards of quality. They may also be able to operate more efficiently by sharing costly equipment and specialized staff. Finally, if the group includes doctors with different specialties, referrals are convenient and your medical record is likely to be comprehensive, incorporating all the specialists' comments.
- *What are the doctor's hours?* Many doctors schedule weekend or evening hours to accommodate patients' work schedules.
- *How does the doctor cover emergencies on nights and weekends?* If a doctor does not have an arrangement with at least one other doctor to share "on call" duties, be wary. Where will you turn when the doctor is out of town, ill, or at a meeting?
- *Does the doctor give advice over the phone to regular patients? Is there a charge for such advice?* Telephone advice can be a great convenience—a partial substitute for the house call most doctors are reluctant to make. With malpractice liability looking them in the eyes, doctors will be careful about phone advice in questionable cases, but most doctors give some advice over the phone. Very few charge to give phone advice as long as patients come in for office visits occasionally and do not call every few days. Some HMOs and large medical groups have phone lines staffed by nurses to give advice on common medical problems.
- *What lab, x-ray, and machine diagnostic tests can be done without your having to go to another office?*
- *What is the usual wait for an appointment for a nonemergency medical problem? For a full physical exam?*
- *What is the charge for a routine followup office visit? For a routine followup hospital visit? For a typical general physical exam?* This may not matter to you, of course, if your plan will be paying, but it will matter if the doctor is not on your plan's provider list or if you will be expected to pay a percentage of the fee.
- *Will the doctor deal with your insurance carrier?* You save time if your doctor will bill your insurance company directly. If you are on Medicare, it is important to know whether the doctor will accept "assignment"—taking the Medicare-approved fee as payment in full.
- *If you are an HMO member: What is the doctor's opinion of your HMO? How does the doctor feel about the HMO's physician compensation system and about its rules on allowing referrals? Is the doctor considering leaving the plan?* You don't want a doctor who resents caring for patients in your plan. And you certainly don't want to choose one who will soon leave the plan and be unavailable to you.

When you have gathered all the information you can from calls to physicians' offices, talks with friends, and other sources, you may want to visit the physician who looks best to you. A visit just to meet a doctor should be inexpensive or free. But some consumers will find a meeting of this kind awkward, and some of the doctors we have interviewed share this feeling. As an alternative, you can schedule a physical exam—although this will be costly unless you are an HMO member.

If you do not feel a relationship with a doctor is immediately necessary, keep your notes on the doctors you have checked and simply call your first choice when a medical problem occurs.

After your first meeting or any subsequent encounter with a doctor, you should feel free to look for a new one if you are not satisfied, and you have a right to your records to pass along to your new doctor. There are a few performance standards any doctor should meet—

- Offers reasonably convenient hours.
- Calls you back the same day if you call with a medical question—within a few minutes if you have left a message that there is an emergency—so long as you don't call much more often than you go in for visits.
- Gives helpful medical advice by phone.
- Generally arranges to see you within a day or two if you call with a new (nonemergency) sickness or injury.
- Generally does not keep you waiting more than 15 minutes past your appointment time before serving you.
- Refers you for specialty care when you think you need it.

- Is thorough and careful and seems to be competent.
- Remembers, or consults records about, your medical history and relevant information you have given before.
- Takes a thorough medical history.
- Listens to you, doesn't interrupt you, and makes you feel comfortable about asking questions.
- Checks your progress, tells you about test results, and follows up with other providers you're referred to.
- Explains what is wrong, what is being done, and what you can expect.
- Tells you about your choices and gets you involved in making decisions about your care.

- Seems personally to care about you and your medical problems.
- Spends enough time with you.
- Gives you helpful advice about ways to stay healthy.
- Gets results as good as you believe you can reasonably expect.

But you will be wise not to shop continually from doctor to doctor. An established relationship with a doctor you like and trust is a real asset. And remember, you don't need a medical genius as your personal doctor. Most of the time any competent doctor will give you the proper medical treatment, and for most of the remaining problems the doctor will know enough to refer you to a more skilled physician for help.

Chapter 8

Getting Good Care in Any Plan

In any health plan, there is much you personally can do to make the system work well for you and to improve the quality of care you receive. Some steps apply mainly in indemnity plans, some in HMOs, and some in all plans.

Learn the Rules

Read carefully through the materials you get when you enroll. In any type of plan, you'll want to find out—

- What types of services are covered and what limitations and exclusions there are.
- What preauthorization is needed—and how to arrange it—prior to hospital admission, surgery, or other expensive services.
- How to file claims.
- What your rights are to have a second opinion paid for by the plan, and how to arrange for one.
- How to call for customer service.
- How to complain about poor service or denial of service.
- How to appeal if you feel your complaint is not handled fairly.

If you are in an HMO, you'll also want to find out—

- How to select a primary care doctor.
- How to set up an appointment.
- How to get a referral for specialty services— whether you can self-refer; what paperwork, if any, you need from your primary care doctor; how often a referral has to be reauthorized.
- Whether there is a special phone number to call for medical advice and when it operates.
- What to do in an emergency—where to go, when to call the plan, what to say to the provider of emergency care.
- Under what circumstances you can get care when you're traveling outside the plan's service area, whether there are certain providers you should use for the service, how soon—and how—you should notify your plan, what you should tell the out-of-area provider.
- How to switch primary care doctors—how quickly it can be done and how frequently.
- What choices of providers you have for specialty care or hospital care—whether you are limited to providers affiliated with your primary care physician.
- Whether there are special programs for exercise, weight loss, stress management, prenatal care, and other prevention activities and how you can find out about them.

If there are rules and procedures you don't understand, ask for clarification from the plan's customer service staff, your insurance agent, or your employer's personnel office.

Keep a File of All the Written Materials You Get From Your Plan

Keep your provider directory (in an HMO or PPO), materials the plan gives you on procedures (for filing claims, switching doctors, getting authorization for hospitalization, etc.), and the contract describing plan benefits and limitations. Also keep your medical bills and all statements of benefits that have been paid. Be sure to carry your plan ID card; you might have to show it to get service from some providers.

Choose a Good Primary Care Doctor

We've discussed this point in Chapter 7. Finding a good primary care doctor is essential to getting good care in any type of plan but especially critical in an HMO, where this doctor will be the "gatekeeper" controlling access to all other services.

Be aware that in many HMOs the primary care doctor you choose will be affiliated with a certain hospital or hospitals and a specific group of specialists, and that these may be the only providers the doctor can refer you to—even though many more providers are listed in the plan's provider directory.

Continually Assess Your Relationship with Your Doctor

Once you've selected a doctor, you should continually assess whether the doctor is giving you the quality of care and service you deserve. Some reasonable performance expectations are listed in Chapter 7.

Being able to communicate and work well with your doctor is critical. Much research has shown that patients with a good relationship to a doctor tend to get more accurate diagnoses, respond better to treatment, put up better with symptoms, and recover more quickly. Certainly, you're more likely to do your part in care—taking medicine and making lifestyle changes—if you understand what is expected of you, why it's important, and what effects you can expect to observe.

If You're Dissatisfied with Your Doctor, Switch

It's not wise to change doctors frequently. You lose the benefit of what you and the doctor have learned about communicating with each other and what the doctor has learned about your medical needs. But if you are dissatisfied, don't delay switching.

In an indemnity plan or PPO and in some HMOs, switching is as easy as making an appointment with a new doctor. In other HMOs, you have to inform the customer service department of your intent to switch and you may have to wait until the first of the next month or even the next open enrollment period. In some network-type HMOs, it's easier to switch to another doctor within the same physician group than to switch to a doctor in another of the HMO's groups.

Even if a plan's standard procedures require you to wait for a period before making a switch, you're likely to be able to move more quickly if you feel a switch is urgent and you ask the plan to make an exception to its rules.

Get Your Medical Records Transferred

Whether you've changed plans and doctors or just changed doctors within a plan, be sure your new doctor gets your medical records from your old doctor. Remember, in many cases your history is the most useful aid in diagnosis—more useful than all the tests and x-rays that can be done now.

If your new doctor isn't interested in getting your old medical records, ask why (it's true that the records may not be easy to read or understand). You may want to get the records to store on your own—or at least be sure the former doctor will save them for many years.

It is also important to pull your records together if you use more than one doctor. For example, if you use a non-HMO doctor when traveling, have your records transferred to your HMO doctor.

Be Sure Your Doctor Takes a Thorough Medical History

If you feel your doctor has not asked about matters that might be important to diagnosing or treating you, volunteer the information. If both of your parents had colon cancer, if your dad had a heart attack at age 40, if you recently had a bout with kidney stones, or if you periodically feel very depressed, let the doctor know.

Find Out About Tests Your Doctor Proposes to Do

Ask your doctor what tests he or she will do during routine visits—mammogram, hemocult to check for blood in your stool, PSA test for prostate cancer, electrocardiogram, sigmoidoscopy to check your rectum and lower colon, cholesterol test, HIV test? Ask why specific tests and not others are given. If there are particular medical problems you're concerned about, ask if there are relevant tests and why they do or don't make sense for you.

There's a lot of debate in the medical field about which routine tests are worth doing for which population groups and how often. There are reasons not to give tests: some are unpleasant, some are costly, some pose risks of complications, and all have the possibility of indicating that you have a problem you really don't have—leading to costly, unpleasant, and possibly dangerous treatment. You should be given an opportunity to express your preferences regarding tests, based on information about each test's pros and cons.

You should learn not only about routine tests given during preventive exams but also about any tests prescribed to check out a specific symptom or medical problem. Ask what each test will tell you that you don't already know, how reliable it is, what the risks and costs are, and whether the results might really make any difference in treatment plans.

Be Sure You Are Told the Results of Exams and Treatment

At the time of a doctor visit, ask when the results will be available and how you'll be told of them. Some doctors tell you nothing unless there is a problem. That approach may leave you wondering long after your doctor has the answers. There's also the risk that phone messages will be lost and you won't realize that a doctor called to give you results. If you know that a doctor is supposed to call and when, you'll be able to check back if the time for your report passes.

Discuss the Results of Exams

When you get test results, ask the doctor to compare them to results from previous tests and ask whether there are changes that might be worth making in your life to improve results. Even if your cholesterol count or your weight is within an acceptable range, for example, is it worse than it was? Enough worse to do something about?

Prepare for Appointments

Before a doctor visit—either a visit to a doctor's office or a visit by the doctor when you are in the hospital—get ready. Think what questions you want answered, what symptoms you've had, what treatments you've been giving yourself or that other providers have been giving you.

Write down your questions and other information to be sure you don't forget to mention something. You might even bring the medications you've been using with you to the doctor's office.

If the doctor seems to be rushing you through your list of items, explain that discussing these matters is important to you and that you think the doctor should give you enough time. You might want to arrange to have a friend with you for the doctor visit to help you push to get through your questions and to help you remember the doctor's responses. You might even take a tape recorder.

Describe Symptoms in Detail

Does the problem occur only after you've just eaten, after you've exercised heavily, when you've been standing for a long time, only when you urinate? What does it feel like? When did you first notice the problem? Your description is a window on what's going on inside—often a better window than all the examining and testing the doctor can do.

If you have fears that you might have a particular medical condition, tell the doctor. This will give the doctor a chance to investigate those concerns or to assure you that they are unfounded.

Find Out About Getting Answers by Phone

Many questions require a visit to the doctor or tests. But some can be resolved based on what you can communicate by phone. Also, a phone call can often help you determine whether a doctor visit is needed—and how soon.

Ask your doctor if there is a nurse you can talk with about questions you may have. And ask what is the best time to reach the doctor by phone.

Ask for a Full Explanation of Your Diagnosis and Treatment Options

When your doctor has had a chance to evaluate your case, be sure you get a full explanation of what he or she has discovered, of the choices you have, and of what you can expect.

What isn't working right? What caused it? What can be done about it now? If it's curable, what can you do differently to avoid a recurrence—

for example, eat differently, exercise differently, sleep differently, sit differently, change jobs, wear a brace?

How sure is the doctor of the diagnosis? What are the other possibilities? What more can be done to confirm the diagnosis? At what cost and what risk?

What are the treatment options? What are the risks and costs? What are the possible benefits in terms of your lifestyle and ability to function? How will you know if the treatment is working? What will you need to report to the doctor?

One of your fundamental rights as a patient is the right to informed consent. If you agree to a treatment—to allow a doctor to act on you with drugs, knives, or other instruments—and it is a treatment you would not have chosen had you better understood your options, the doctor's actions really amount to an assault. That's why responsible doctors understand the importance of trying to answer all your questions.

Ask About Specialists

If your doctor refers you to a specialist, ask why a specialist is needed and why that particular specialist was chosen. What is known about his or her expertise and experience with your type of case? Is this the only specialist of this type that your primary doctor is able to refer you to under his or her arrangements with your health plan?

What should you expect the specialist to do? How will your primary care doctor remain involved in your care?

If you are not referred to a specialist, ask why not. What extra expertise might a specialist bring to the case?

Remember that some plans have physician compensation schemes that penalize—or reward—a doctor for making referrals to specialists.

Ask About Medication

If medication is recommended, ask why that particular medication. What benefits is it expected to have? How soon? What are the possible side effects and what should you do if you experience them? How should you take the medication—for example, with meals, at bedtime? Can you take it even though you're taking other medications? What should you do if you forget to take a dose? Will the medication limit your capacity to drive, work, or do other activities?

Ask About Hospitalization

If hospitalization is not recommended, ask why not. Hospitals are expensive and health plans are interested in cutting costs. If a plan pays its doctors by an arrangement that gives less income when patients are hospitalized, you want to be sure the financial incentives are not causing you to get too little care.

On the other hand, if hospitalization is recommended, ask why. Could the case be handled on an outpatient basis?

Hospitals are dangerous places. In a recent report, the Institute of Medicine of the National Academy of Sciences summarized evidence from the two major studies on just how dangerous: "the results of these two studies imply that at least 44,000 and perhaps as many as 98,000 Americans die in hospitals each year as a result of medical errors." And there are many additional cases where hospital or doctor negligence slows recovery or leads to short-term or long-term disability. So you don't want to go into a hospital unnecessarily. But in many health plans that pay doctors on a fee-for-service basis, the doctor may have a financial incentive to put you in a hospital where extensive and expensive services can be performed.

Also, be sure to ask why a particular hospital was chosen. Is it the only hospital to which your doctor is allowed to refer under arrangements with your health plan?

How complicated is your case? Does it require sophisticated hospital staff or advanced equipment? What are the risks of complications? Will it be important to have close monitoring and quick access to medical staff and equipment at all times? If the case is complicated, a major teaching hospital might be best.

Is your required treatment one for which special training or frequent experience is important? Are there certain hospitals where the staffs have more skill, more experience, or higher success rates than others with this treatment? In many types of cases—such as open heart surgery—research has shown that hospitals that treat a greater number of patients generally have better results.

Get a Second Opinion

If your doctor recommends hospitalization or other treatment that will be expensive, risky, or burdensome, get a second opinion. In such cases, most doctors will encourage second opinions. Most plans will be glad to pay, since the second opinion may lead to a recommendation of less care—and less cost.

If your doctor recommends against certain types of care that you know are available or if you are not confident in your doctor's conclusions or satisfied with the progress of your case, you might want a second opinion to consider more or different care. In an indemnity plan or PPO, you can arrange for a second opinion on your own and the plan will generally pay for it. In an HMO, your doctor will have to refer you for the second opinion in order for the plan to pay. Since the second opinion might lead to more care, there may be some resistance to authorizing it. If you think a second opinion is justified, insist on one. If the first and second opinions are in conflict or for some other reason you're still not confident in the conclusions, insist on a third opinion.

If possible, get your second opinion from an entirely independent doctor. If a surgeon who has recommended surgery refers you to another surgeon for a second opinion, it will be difficult for the second doctor to recommend against the advice (and the economic interests) of the first. To find a doctor to use for a second opinion, you can ask friends and co-workers for recommendations, contact a medical school, or ask for a referral from a well-regarded hospital. If you read up on your type of case—especially if it is of a type that is being actively researched at certain medical centers—you may come upon names of leading specialists who might be available for advice. You can also find good doctors for this purpose in our *Guide to Top Doctors*, which you can order for $19.95 from Checkbook's Doctor Guide, 733 15th Street, NW, Suite 820, Washington, DC 20005, or subscribe to online at *www.checkbook.org*.

You'll have more flexibility in choosing an independent doctor if you are in an indemnity plan or PPO than if you are in an HMO. In an HMO, your primary care doctor is likely to refer you to another participating doctor with whom he or she has regular contact.

To keep down the cost and time required for a second opinion, have your first doctor send copies of your medical records, x-rays, and lab results to the second opinion doctor. This is standard procedure.

Don't assume that because yours is a straightforward, uncomplicated case there is nothing to learn and there are no decisions to be made. In most cases, there are choices.

This point is brought home by studies done by Dartmouth Medical School researchers and others, looking at variations in medical practice in common types of cases across similar geographic areas. One of these studies found, for example, that about 75 percent of the elderly men in one Maine town had undergone prostate surgery, compared with fewer than 25 percent of men the same age in an adjacent town. Similar variations have been found in rates of hysterectomies, caesarean sections, and other common procedures. Significantly, studies generally find no evidence that such medical practice differences result in differences in the health status of the affected populations.

The implication is that big differences in the ways patients are treated result from differences in the beliefs and customs of different physicians in different communities—possibly influenced by the need to generate fees and not necessarily based on sound evidence of likely benefits to the patient. Even in a common type of case, you can't assume that a physician's standard recommendation is the best option for you.

Do Your Own Medical Research

Asking doctors questions is one way to learn. But you'll learn more—and have a better opportunity to grasp the information at your own pace—if you seek out published materials from other sources.

You can use available libraries. At any major public library, you can ask for general consumer-oriented medical literature or for medical texts. For more in-depth information, you can use a medical school library. These libraries may also be able to help you find support groups and organizations that regularly provide information on your type of medical problem.

You can also find an enormous amount of information online. You can use any major search engine to find information on a disease, test, or treatment. But be careful about the information you use. Inaccurate information can find its way to the Web just as easily as reliable information. And much of what you find on the Web is paid for by commercial interests, with resulting biases. A Federal government website with basic information is *www.healthfinder.gov*. A valuable resource for a wide variety of information is the website of the National Library of Medicine or the Federal government's National Institutes of Health at *www.nlm.nih.gov*. In addition to other information available at this website, you can locate the most authoritative articles on any medical subject. You can read summaries of many articles online and then order copies, for a fee, from a participating medical library.

Complain If Necessary

If you've had a hard time getting a question about your coverage answered, your records weren't transferred as requested when you switched doctors, payment on a claim was delayed, a plan doctor was rude to you, or you've experienced any other problem that you couldn't resolve directly with the personnel involved, call or write your plan's member services department.

Your plan should respond promptly. If you are not satisfied with the response, you can file a formal grievance. Read your plan's contract to find out the grievance procedure.

Appeal If Necessary

If you feel your plan has unjustifiably refused to pay for a doctor visit you made because you had chest pain while away on a trip, refused to authorize a new form of chemotherapy because the plan considers the treatment experimental, refused to refer you to a leading hospital for unusual heart surgery, or in some other way denied you care or coverage you think you should have had, see if your employer's benefits manager or your insurance agent can help reverse the decision. If not, appeal. In many plans, your contract sets out a member appeal process. In many HMOs, there is an appeals committee that includes members, and you will be given a chance to attend a hearing. You should get a written decision. If you are not satisfied, you can turn to a state regulatory agency or take the plan to court (or to arbitration if the plan has agreed to that option).

Follow Plan Procedures

You're less likely to have disputes with your plan if you strictly follow required procedures.

For example, if you are in an HMO, be sure not to use nonplan doctors when you are traveling outside the plan's service area unless your case meets the plan's definition of urgent. If you've had a headache for two weeks and decide to see a doctor about it on the first day of your trip, you're likely to have a problem with your plan. Similarly, if your plan requires preauthorization of surgery, be sure to get the authorization.

Appendix A

About the Doctor and Member Surveys

For you to know how much weight to put on the data in the Plan Ratings table in Chapter 4, it is useful to have some background on the survey methods, strengths, and limitations.

Our Survey of Doctors

We mailed questionnaires to approximately 260,000 doctors. The list included, to the extent we were able, all actively practicing doctors, other than doctors still in training, in the largest metropolitan areas in the U.S. Approximately 20,000 responded. You will notice that doctor survey data are available on the Plan Ratings table only for plans that serve the 53 largest metropolitan statistical areas (MSAs) or primary metropolitan statistical areas (PMSAs) and a few other populous areas, which for the most part, are adjacent to the 53 areas.

The survey had several sections. In one section, we asked the doctors to name for us the one or two specialists, in each of 35 specialty fields, whom they "would consider most desirable for care of a loved one." The results from that part of the survey are one element in another *Consumers' CHECKBOOK* publication, our *Guide to Top Doctors*. In a second section, we asked the doctors to rate hospitals in their communities. The results from that section contributed, along with much other data, to the hospital ratings in our *Consumers' Guide to Hospitals*. A third section asked the doctors to rate the HMOs they were familiar with from a list of HMOs in their communities.

The questionnaire instructed the doctors: "Based on all that you know from your own experience and from HMOs' reputations among your peers, please rate all the HMOs that you can on the list in the table below. Evaluate each HMO relative to your opinion of what constitutes a high professional standard of care within an HMO." While we invited ratings of HMOs with which doctors had no history of affiliation, we asked the doctors to indicate their affiliation, if any, with each HMO—

- Currently affiliated with HMO
- Not currently affiliated, but have been affiliated within the past two years
- No affiliation with HMO within the past two years

On the Plan Ratings table, we report only ratings given by doctors who said they were currently affiliated or had been affiliated within the past two years with the HMO they were rating.

We asked 10 questions about each HMO. These questions were developed and refined based on a number of other questionnaires we have had the opportunity to review. In particular, we have reviewed questionnaires and tens of thousands of responses from surveys many health plans themselves use to learn about doctors' opinions. The specific questions we asked addressed issues that matter to consumers—not matters that would be of special interest only to doctors, such as the fee schedules the plans use to pay doctors.

The doctors rated the plans on a five-point scale: "poor," "fair," "good," "very good," or "excellent." The Plan Ratings table shows the percentage of "good," "very good," or "excellent" responses for each question.

Several cautions need to be taken into account in using the doctor survey data:

- Most of the doctors responding currently worked for the plans they were rating. Doctors might have financial reasons for rating favorably a plan that might steer patients to them or that might, if rated favorably, eventually have more money to pay its doctors. The concern is that some plans might have stronger relationships with responding doctors than other plans have. This is especially a concern with the relatively small number of HMOs that have doctors who work only for them—plans that have their own clinics or doctor groups.

- The mix of responding doctors might be different from plan to plan. For example, for a plan that has an unusually large number of specialists relative to primary care doctors, the ratings on the Plan Ratings table will be disproportionately from specialists. Specialists tend to give plans lower ratings than primary care physicians give them. Also, some plans might have older physicians than others have, and older doctors tend to give somewhat lower ratings than younger doctors. We considered adjusting the results for these and other physician characteristics but did not do so because the adjustments would have small effects, rarely affecting a plan's scores by more than two or three percentage points.

  There are also other characteristics of doctors that appear to be related to plan scores and vary from plan to plan, but for which we could not adjust without possibly adjusting away real plan performance differences. One such characteristic is disaffiliation with a plan within the past two years. Recently disaffiliated doctors tend to give lower ratings than currently affiliated doctors. If the disaffiliation was not voluntary on the part of the doctor—for example, if it occurred simply because the plan changed its service area—it might make sense to adjust for this doctor characteristic. But some disaffiliations might have taken place because doctors thought plans were providing poor care, and it would not be appropriate to adjust away that effect. Also, the data have not been adjusted for regional differences in attitudes and expectations among rating doctors. There is some evidence that doctors in different regions might have different standards, but it is also possible that plans in some regions are simply better than plans in other regions. Fortunately this regional issue won't lessen the value of the data for most users, since you probably will be comparing plans only in a single region.

- Some doctors may not know much about plans. This is especially true in parts of the country where the plans typically contract with physician groups rather than with individual doctors and where plan quality improvement programs and programs to restrict services are generally implemented by plans' communications with the groups, which in turn communicate with the doctors. Even where doctors contract directly with plans, often it is the office staff, not the doctor, that has most of the plan contact. But it seems likely that doctors will be aware of any significant quality improvement programs; it is, after all, the doctors who must implement such programs. And it seems likely that doctors will be aware of any unusual restrictions on care a plan imposes since it will often be the doctor's patterns of care that are disrupted.

- The plan the doctors were rating might not be exactly the same entity you would consider joining. The survey asked the doctors to rate HMOs. Some HMO companies have various plan models—with and without a point of service option, for example, or with and without a requirement that members go through a gatekeeper primary care physician in order to see a specialist. The doctors probably could not separate out their experiences with an HMO company to report only on the basic HMO model. Even if they did, that might not be the model you are considering.

- Survey respondents may be different from nonrespondents. It is often speculated that respondent ratings of any service will be lower than nonrespondent ratings. We did not do follow-up surveying to test this hypothesis. But this nonresponse bias is unlikely to have had an effect on the relative rankings of plans unless some plans had lower response rates than others or the ratings of nonrespondents versus respondents are more negative for some plans than for others. It is worth noting that the decision to respond to the survey was probably not driven for most doctors by the desire to rate HMOs; the sections of the questionnaire that called for recommendations of physicians and ratings of hospitals came first and took up more space on the questionnaire.

- Differences in plans' scores might be explained by chance alone. A plan might have simply had the bad luck that the doctors who liked the plan didn't happen to respond in as great numbers as doctors who disliked the plan. This is a bigger concern if the number of raters for a plan is small. The Plan Ratings table reports the number of doctors who rated each plan, so you can take that into account in deciding how much confidence to put in the plan's scores. We did not report physician survey results for any plan that was rated by fewer than 25 doctors. For a plan that was rated by 25 doctors and received 40 percent favorable ratings, you can be 95 percent confident that its score wouldn't have been more than 20 percentage points higher or lower if the sample of respondents had simply been larger. For a plan rated by 100 doctors, you can be 95 percent confident that its score wouldn't have been more than 10 percentage points higher or lower if the sample of respondents had simply been larger.

- The plan's performance in the service area rated by the doctors might not be the same as its performance in the specific area where you live. The surveyed doctors were rating each plan's performance within a metropolitan area that often didn't correspond to the plan's full service area. Wherever possible, we pooled physician ratings for several different metropolitan areas—for example, San Diego, Los Angeles and Orange counties, San Bernardino and Riverside counties, the San Francisco Bay Area, and the Sacramento area for some California plans—but even the pooled data might not cover the plan's entire service area. Even if the doctors' ratings were representative of a plan's entire service area, it's possible that the plan performs better or worse in the specific subpart of its service area where you live.

- There might have been some problems matching the doctor survey data with the data from the other sources and with the name listed on the Plan Ratings table. The doctors rated plans according to the plan names we listed on the questionnaire. But plan names change and the

same plan might have several different variants of its name. Beginning on page 86 is a list that tells you which names used in the doctor survey were matched up with which names on the Plan Ratings table.

The Survey of Plan Members

The survey of health plan members was done using a questionnaire developed with funding and leadership from the U.S. Agency for Healthcare Research and Quality (AHRQ). Except for minor variations in a few plans (noted in the footnotes for the Plan Ratings table) in Florida, all of the surveys were carried out using a set of procedures dictated by the National Committee for Quality Assurance (NCQA). These procedures called for the following sequence of five mailings: presurvey postcard, questionnaire with cover letter, reminder postcard, second questionnaire with cover letter to nonrespondents, second reminder postcard. For nonrespondents to these mailed attempts, six attempts were made to complete the survey by phone. The initial sample size for each plan was 1,500 and response rates were generally in the 45 percent range, yielding about 650 to 700 responses.

Each plan was required to have its survey carried out by an independent survey research firm. The plan could choose the survey firm, but the survey firm had to be trained and certified by NCQA, and NCQA monitored the survey process. Each plan supplied its survey firm its entire list of eligible members and the survey firm drew a random sample of these members to survey. The list of eligible members was checked by an independent audit firm to assure that it was complete.

The surveyed members scored the firms using several different scales. For the items on the Plan Ratings table, the following scales were used—

- Zero to 10 scale. The Plan Ratings table reports the percent of respondents who rated the plans "8," "9," or "10" for—
    ➡ Overall rating of plan
    ➡ Overall health care
    ➡ Personal doctors
    ➡ Specialist doctors
- "Big problem," "Small problem," or "Not a problem" scale. The Plan Ratings table reports the percent of respondents who rated plans "Not a problem" for "Plan's customer service." The table also reports the percent of respondents who said they did not have any problems getting referrals, tests, and treatment; and the percent of respondents who said they had had a "Big problem" getting referrals, tests, and treatment.
- "Never," "Sometimes," "Usually," or "Always" scale. The Plan Ratings table reports the percent of respondents who rated plans in the two most favorable categories for—
    ➡ Getting care quickly
    ➡ How well doctors communicate
    ➡ Claims processing

As with the doctor survey data, several cautions need to be considered when using the member survey data:

- If you look just at the overall ratings of each plan, you might not spot serious problems. One can imagine a plan having restrictive policies that routinely deny members life-saving but expensive therapy while at the same time having an excellent newsletter and a special arrangement to get members a big price break on memberships at local health and fitness clubs. Since only a few members each year need expensive life-saving treatment, their negative ratings of the plan would not have much effect on the plan's overall percent of favorable ratings, while the favorable ratings from the many members who might enjoy the newsletter or the fitness club discount would have give the plan a big lift in its overall percentage of favorable ratings. The ratings on the table for "Big" problem getting needed referrals/ tests/treatment might help you spot serious care denials. (Members who had a "big problem" also were more likely than other categories of members to give plans a score of "0" on the zero to 10 scale for overall rating of plan.) But it is important to keep in mind the theoretical possibility that even a plan with such egregious approval policies that it *killed* one percent of its members each year could do enough customer-friendly things in less serious circumstances to come out with an average or better score on most or all survey questions.

- There may be plan-to-plan differences in the characteristics of the survey respondents, and some plans might have been rated by respondents who are more or less difficult to please than other plans' respondents. In extensive analyses of survey data from hundreds of plans, we have found that differences in age, education level, and health status account for significant differences in plan scores. The scores reported on the Plan Ratings table have not been adjusted for these or other respondent characteristics, but the effects of adjustment would be fairly small. Very few plans' scores would change more than two percentage points if the scores were adjusted. Among plans that would be in the top quarter of all plans based on actual scores, only about 10 percent would cease to be in the top quarter if the scores were adjusted.

- The members who responded to the survey might have had different opinions and experiences with the plans than nonrespondents. Our review of the data indicates that younger members and men, especially men under age 35, are less likely to respond than older members and women. Young males also tend to give somewhat lower ratings than older members of either gender. Fortunately, with roughly half the sampled members responding for most plans, the respondents do at least represent a substantial portion of members. And there is some evidence that scores would not have changed much if an even larger portion of members had responded. We have done special studies in which an extra survey mailing was done, increasing the number of respondents by 10 to 15 percent, and these extra respondents on average rated their plans only two to three percentage points lower than earlier respondents.

- Differences in plans' scores might be explained by chance alone. As with the doctor survey, with the member survey a plan might have simply had the bad luck that the persons who liked it least happened to respond. But this is less of a concern with members than with doctors because the number of surveyed members who responded was relatively large—more than 600 respondents for most plans for most questions. For a plan rated by 600 members, you can be 95 percent confident that its score wouldn't have been more than four percentage points higher or lower than that reported on the Plan Ratings table if the sample of respondents had simply been larger.

- Some differences in plan scores result from differences in the mode—mail versus telephone—by which the respondents were surveyed. Some plans reached a relatively large portion of their respondents by mail; others got relatively few by mail and more through telephone followup. (Many plans don't have phone numbers for many of their members, so it is difficult for the surveyors to reach members by phone.) We have done analyses indicating that telephone respondents rate plans differently from the way mail respondents rate them. The overall rating of plans tends to be about seven percentage points higher for telephone respondents than for mail respondents. We even have data on members who responded twice to the same

survey, having been reached by phone before the Postal Service delivered their returned mail questionnaire. On the "Overall rating of plan" question with the zero to 10 rating scale, the ratings given by these mail-and-phone respondents were about twice as likely to be higher by phone than mail as they were to be higher by mail than by phone. Fortunately, since few plans got large portions of their responses by phone, the effects of mode differences on plan-to-plan differences in scores on the Plan Ratings table is rarely more than two or three percentage points.

- Scores might have been affected by use of the Internet. NCQA allowed plans to use an "enhanced" survey procedure in which members were offered the option to complete the survey over the Internet. A substantial number of plans did so. Special test data we have analyzed indicates that within the same plan, members who are offered the option to rate the plan via the Internet and choose to do so tend to rate it nearly 15 percentage points lower than members who are given only the mail and phone survey options. Fortunately, most plans that offered surveyed members the Internet survey option actually got few responses via the Internet, so the effect of those responses on plan scores was probably less than one percentage point.

- Scores might have been affected by the language of response. NCQA allowed surveyors the option of sending both an English-language and a Spanish-language questionnaire to each surveyed member. Some plans with substantial percentages of members who had expressed a Spanish-language preference took this approach, but others did not. Our analysis indicates that members of the same plan rating the plan on the Spanish-language questionnaire tended to give ratings about 20 percentage points higher than members using the English-language version. This effect is not likely to explain many differences on the Plan Ratings table, however, because very few plans adopted the two-questionnaire approach, and even in those plans, few members used the Spanish-language questionnaire.

- Scores might have been affected by a plan's decision on the specific product line to survey. Some plans surveyed only their basic HMO members or only their POS members. Others surveyed both those members from both lines of business, HMO and POS. Among members of the same plan, POS members are about two to three percentage points less likely than basic HMO members to give high ratings to the overall plan. We have noted next to each plan name on the Plan Ratings table whether the member survey, accreditation review, and direct measures of care apply only to a plan's HMO business or only to POS business. If a plan's name doesn't have the notation "HMO" or "POS" in aprentheses next to it, the data are for the plan's combined HMO and POS business.

- The plan variant that the surveyed members rated might not be the same plan variant you are considering. If the member ratings on the Plan Ratings table were for a basic HMO and you are considering a POS option or an HMO without a gatekeeper requirement also offered by the same organization, the ratings on the table won't be strictly applicable to your situation. We have not attempted to identify the specific plan design variant the surveyed members were rating.

- The plan's performance in your specific geographic area may not be the same as in other areas from which some or most of the surveyed members were drawn.

The cumulative effects of all these considerations might have substantial impact on the extent to which the information on the Plan Ratings table allows you to draw sharp distinctions among plans. But these data are the best available and should help you substantially improve your odds of choosing a plan where you will get good care and service.

Details on How We Matched Up Data

The following table shows, for each listing on the Plan Ratings table that begins on page 22: the plan's name as listed in the source of the plan's member satisfaction data, codes for the regions from which physician survey data were used, and the plan's name as listed on the physicians survey for each area. On page 93 are a key to the region codes for the physician survey and a description of which counties we surveyed for each region.

Plan	Plan's name as listed in member satisfaction data source	Doctors survey area(s) and how plan's name appeared on survey(s)
Arizona		
Aetna U.S. Healthcare (Southern and western Arizona)	Aetna U.S. Healthcare, Inc. - Arizona	PHOEN: Aetna U.S. Healthcare
BlueCross BlueShield of Arizona (All or most of Arizona)	No data	PHOEN: BlueCross BlueShield of Arizona
CIGNA HealthCare of Arizona (Parts of Arizona)	CIGNA HealthCare of Arizona, Inc.	PHOEN: CIGNA HealthCare of Arizona
Health Net of Arizona (HMO) (Most of Arizona)	Health Net of Arizona, Inc. (HMO)	PHOEN: Health Net of Arizona
Humana Health Plans (HMO) (Southern and western Arizona)	Humana Health Plan, Inc. (Arizona) (HMO)	PHOEN: Humana Health Plan
Mayo Health Plan Arizona (Phoenix area)	No data	PHOEN: Mayo Health Plan Arizona
PacifiCare of Arizona (HMO) (Phoenix and Tuscon areas)	PacifiCare of Arizona, Inc. (HMO)	PHOEN: PacifiCare of Arizona
UnitedHealthcare of Arizona (All or most of Arizona)	No data	PHOEN: UnitedHealthcare of Arizona
Arkansas		
Aetna U.S. Healthcare (Crittenden County)	Prudential HealthCare Plan, Inc., A Member Company of Aetna U.S. Healthcare - Memphis	No data
HealthLink (HMO) (Little Rock area and parts of Northern Arkansas)	HealthLink, Inc. (HMO)	STLOU: HealthLink HMO
HealthLink (POS) (Little Rock area and parts of Northern Arkansas)	HealthLink, Inc. (POS)	STLOU: HealthLink HMO
UnitedHealthcare of Arkansas (Most of Arkansas)	United HealthCare of Arkansas, Inc.	No data
California		
Aetna U.S. Healthcare (Northern California)	Aetna U.S. Healthcare of California Inc. - North	SFRAN: Aetna U.S. Healthcare
Aetna U.S. Healthcare (Most of Southern California)	Aetna U.S. Healthcare of California - South	LOSAN: Aetna U.S. Healthcare of CA; RIVER: Aetna U.S. Healthcare
Aetna U.S. Healthcare (San Diego County)	Aetna U.S. Healthcare of California - San Diego	SDIEG: Aetna U.S. Healthcare
Blue Cross of California/California Care (Most or all of California)	Blue Cross of California	LOSAN: CaliforniaCare; SDIEG: CaliforniaCare; SFRAN: CaliforniaCare; RIVER: CaliforniaCare; SACRA: CaliforniaCare
Blue Shield of California (Most of California)	Blue Shield of California	LOSAN: Blue Shield of CA Access+HMO; SDIEG: Blue Shield of CA Access + HMO; SFRAN: Blue Shield of CA Access + HMO; RIVER: Blue Shield of CA Access+HMO; SACRA: Blue Shield of CA Access + HMO
CIGNA HealthCare of California (Most of California)	CIGNA HealthCare of California, Inc.	LOSAN: CIGNA HealthCare of CA; SDIEG: CIGNA HealthCare of California; SFRAN: CIGNA HealthCare of California; RIVER: CIGNA HealthCare of California; SACRA: CIGNA HealthCare of California
Health Net of California (Most of California)	Health Net	LOSAN: Health Net; SDIEG: Health Net; SFRAN: Health Net; RIVER: Health Net; SACRA: Health Net
HP of the Redwoods (HMO) (Lake, Marin, Mendocino, Sonoma)	Health Plan of the Redwoods (HMO)	SFRAN: Health Plan of the Redwoods
InterValley HP (LA, Orange, Riverside, San Bernardino, Ventura counties)	No data	LOSAN: Inter Valley Health Plan; RIVER: Inter Valley Health Plan
Kaiser Permanente California (HMO) (Northern California)	Kaiser Foundation Health Plan, Inc. - Northern California (HMO)	SFRAN: Kaiser Foundation Health Plan; SACRA: Kaiser Foundation Health Plan
Kaiser Permanente California (HMO) (Southern California)	Kaiser Foundation Health Plan Inc. - Southern California (HMO)	LOSAN: Kaiser Foundation HP-So. CA; SDIEG: Kaiser Foundation Health Plan; RIVER: Kaiser Foundation Health Plan
Lifeguard (HMO) (Northern California)	Lifeguard, Inc (HMO)	SFRAN: Lifeguard; SACRA: Lifeguard
One Health Plan of CA (Bay Area, Fresno, Sacramento, and So. CA)	No data	LOSAN: One Health Plan of California; SDIEG: One Health Plan of California; SFRAN: One Health Plan of California; RIVER: One Health Plan of California; SACRA: One Health Plan of California

Plan	Plan's name as listed in member satisfaction data source	Doctors survey area(s) and how plan's name appeared on survey(s)
PacifiCare of California (Most of California)	PacifiCare of California	LOSAN: PacifiCare of California; SDIEG: PacifiCare of California; SFRAN: PacifiCare of California; RIVER: PacifiCare of California; SACRA: PacifiCare of California
Sharp Health Plan (HMO) (San Diego)	Sharp Health Plan (HMO)	SDIEG: Sharp Health Plan
UHP Healthcare (Los Angeles area)	No data	LOSAN: UHP Healthcare; RIVER: UHP Healthcare
Universal Care (HMO) (Southern California)	Universal Care (HMO)	LOSAN: Universal Care; SDIEG: Universal Care; RIVER: Universal Care
Western Health Advantage (HMO) (Sacramento area)	Western Health Advantage (HMO)	SACRA: Western Health Advantage
Colorado		
Aetna U.S. Healthcare (Front Range area)	Aetna U.S. Healthcare, Inc. - Colorado	DENVR: Aetna U.S. Healthcare
CIGNA HealthCare of Colorado (Front Range area)	CIGNA HealthCare of Colorado	DENVR: CIGNA HealthCare of Colorado
Community Health Plan of the Rockies (Front Range area)	No data	DENVR: Community HP of the Rockies
Denver Health Medical Plan (HMO) (Denver)	Denver Health Medical Plan, Inc. (HMO)	No data
HMO Colorado (Most or all of Colorado)	HMO Colorado	DENVR: HMO Colorado (Anthem BCBS)
Kaiser Permanente Colorado (Denver and Colorado Springs areas)	Kaiser Permanente, Colorado	DENVR: Kaiser Foundation HP of Colorado
One Health Plan of Colorado (Front Range area)	No data	DENVR: One Health Plan of Colorado
PacifiCare of Colorado (Front Range area)	PacifiCare of Colorado, Inc.	DENVR: PacifiCare of Colorado
Rocky Mountain HMO (Most of CO)	Rocky Mountain HMO	DENVR: Rocky Mountain HMO
UnitedHealthcare of Colorado (HMO) (Front Range area)	UnitedHealthcare of Colorado (HMO)	DENVR: UnitedHealthcare of Colorado
Connecticut		
Aetna U.S. Healthcare (All or most of Connecticut)	Aetna U.S. Healthcare Inc. - Connecticut	FAIRF: Aetna U.S. Healthcare; HARTF: Aetna U.S. Healthcare
Anthem Blue Cross and Blue Shield (All or most of Connecticut)	Anthem Blue Cross and Blue Shield - Connecticut	FAIRF: Anthem BC/BS of CT (BlueCare); HARTF: Anthem BC/BS of CT (BlueCare)
CIGNA HealthCare of Connecticut (All of Connecticut)	CIGNA HealthCare of Connecticut	FAIRF: CIGNA HealthCare of CT; HARTF: CIGNA HealthCare of Connecticut
ConnectiCare (All or most of Connecticut)	ConnectiCare, Inc.	FAIRF: ConnectiCare; HARTF: ConnectiCare
First Choice Health Plan (All or most of Connecticut)	No data	FAIRF: First Choice Health Plan
Health Net of the Northeast (All or most of Connecticut)	Health Net, Inc.	FAIRF: Health Net (formerly PHS); HARTF: Health Net (formerly PHS)
Health New England (Northern CT)	Health New England, Inc.	No data
HMO New England (All or most of Connecticut)	No data	FAIRF: HMO New England; HARTF: HMO New England
MedSpan Health Options (All or most of Connecticut)	No data	FAIRF: MedSpan Health Options; HARTF: MedSpan Health Options
Oxford Health Plans (All or most of Connecticut)	Oxford Health Plans - Connecticut	FAIRF: Oxford Health Plans of CT; HARTF: Oxford Health Plans of CT
UnitedHealthcare of New York (Fairfield County)	United HealthCare of New York, Inc.	NYORK: UnitedHealthcare of New York; FAIRF: UnitedHealthcare
Delaware		
Aetna U.S. Healthcare (Northern DE)	Aetna U.S. Healthcare Southern New Jersey	PHILA: Aetna U.S. Healthcare (NJ)
AmeriHealth HMO of Delaware (All of Delaware)	AmeriHealth HMO, Inc. Delaware	PHILA: AmeriHealth HMO
BlueCross BlueShield of Delaware (All of Delaware)	Blue Cross Blue Shield of Delaware, Inc., A Care First Company	No data
CIGNA HealthCare of Delaware (All of Delaware)	CIGNA HealthCare of Delaware, Inc.	PHILA: CIGNA HealthCare of Delaware
Coventry Health Care (All of Delaware)	Coventry Health Care of Delaware, Inc.	PHILA: Coventry Health Care of Delaware; WASDC: Coventry Health Care of Delaware
Delmarva Health Plan (All of Delaware)	Delmarva Health Plan, Inc.	No data

Plan	Plan's name as listed in member satisfaction data source	Doctors survey area(s) and how plan's name appeared on survey(s)
Keystone Health Plan East (All or most of Delaware)	Keystone Health Plan East, Inc.	PHILA: Keystone Health Plan East; JERSE: Keystone Health Plan East
Optimum Choice (All of Delaware)	Optimum Choice, Inc.	WASDC: Optimum Choice; BALTI: Optimum Choice; NORFO: Optimum Choice

District of Columbia

Plan	Plan's name as listed	Doctors survey area(s)
Aetna U.S. Healthcare (District of Columbia)	Aetna U.S. Healthcare Inc. - Maryland, DC and Virginia	WASDC: Aetna U.S. Healthcare; BALTI: Aetna U.S. Healthcare
Capital Care/CareFirst (District of Columbia)	Capital Care, Inc.	WASDC: CapitalCare; BALTI: CareFirst BlueCross BlueShield
CIGNA HealthCare Mid-Atlantic (District of Columbia)	CIGNA HealthCare Mid-Atlantic, Inc.	WASDC: CIGNA HealthCare Mid-Atlantic; BALTI: CIGNA HealthCare Mid-Atlantic
Kaiser Foundation Health Plan Mid-Atlantic States (HMO) (DC)	Kaiser Foundation Health Plan of the Mid-Atlantic States, Inc. (HMO)	WASDC: Kaiser Foundation Health Plan; BALTI: Kaiser Foundation Health Plan
M.D. IPA (District of Columbia)	MD - Individual Practice Association, Inc.	WASDC: M.D. IPA; BALTI: M.D. IPA; NORFO: M.D. IPA
Optimum Choice (District of Columbia)	Optimum Choice, Inc.	WASDC: Optimum Choice; BALTI: Optimum Choice; NORFO: Optimum Choice
Preferred Health Network (District of Columbia)	The Preferred Health Network	WASDC: PHN-HMO (Preferred Hlth Netwk); BALTI: PHN-HMO
UnitedHealthcare of the Mid-Atlantic (HMO) (District of Columbia)	United Healthcare of the Mid-Atlantic (HMO)	WASDC: UnitedHealthcare Mid-Atlantic; BALTI: UnitedHealthcare Mid-Atlantic

Florida

Plan	Plan's name as listed	Doctors survey area(s)
Aetna U.S. Healthcare (Most of Florida)	Aetna U.S. Healthcare, Inc. - Florida	SOFLA: Aetna U.S. Healthcare; TAMPA: Aetna U.S. Healthcare; ORLAN: Aetna U.S. Healthcare; FTMEY: Aetna U.S. Healthcare
AvMed (HMO) (Most of Florida)	AvMed Health Plan (HMO)	SOFLA: AvMed Health Plan; TAMPA: AvMed Health Plan; ORLAN: AvMed Health Plan; FTMEY: AvMed Health Plan
Beacon Health Plans (South Florida)	Beacon Health Plans	SOFLA: Beacon Health Plans; TAMPA: Beacon Health Plans; ORLAN: Beacon Health Plans
Capital Health Plan (HMO) (Tallahassee area)	Capital Group Health Services of Florida, Inc. dba Capital Health Plan (HMO)	No data
CIGNA HealthCare of Florida (Most of Florida)	CIGNA Health Care	SOFLA: CIGNA HealthCare of Florida; TAMPA: CIGNA HealthCare of Florida; ORLAN: CIGNA HealthCare of Florida; FTMEY: CIGNA HealthCare of Florida
Florida 1st Health Plans (Central Florida)	Florida 1st Health Plan	TAMPA: Florida 1st Health Plan; FTMEY: Florida 1st Health Plan
Florida Health Care Plans (Flagler and Volusia counties)	Florida Health Care Plan	ORLAN: Florida Health Care Plan
Foundation Health (South, central, and western Florida)	Foundation Health, a Florida Health Plan, Inc.	SOFLA: Foundation Health; TAMPA: Foundation Health; ORLAN: Foundation Health
Health First Health Plans (HMO) (Brevard and Indian River counties)	Health First Health Plans, Inc. (HMO)	ORLAN: Health First HMO
Health Options (Central, eastern, and southern Florida)	Health Options Inc. - South	SOFLA: Health Options; ORLAN: Health Options
Health Options (Northern and western Florida)	Health Options Inc. - North	TAMPA: Health Options; FTMEY: Health Options
Healthplan Southeast (Gainesville, Ocala, Pensacola, Tallahassee)	HealthPlan Southeast	No data
Humana Health Plans (HMO) (Central Florida)	Humana Medical Plan, Inc. - Central Florida (HMO)	ORLAN: Humana Medical Plan
Humana Health Plans (HMO) (Northern Florida)	Humana Medical Plan, Inc. - North Florida (HMO)	No data
Humana Health Plans (HMO) (South Florida)	Humana Medical Plan, Inc. - South Florida (HMO)	SOFLA: Humana Medical Plan; FTMEY: Humana Medical Plan
Humana Health Plans (HMO) (Tampa Bay area)	Humana Medical Plan, Inc. (Tampa) (HMO)	TAMPA: Humana Medical Plan
JMH Health Plan (Broward and Miami-Dade counties)	JMH Health Plan	SOFLA: JMH Health Plan
Neighborhood Health Partnership (South Florida)	Neighborhood Health Partnership, Inc.	SOFLA: Neighborhood Health Partnership
One Health Plan (Fort Myers, Orlando, South Florida, Tampa Bay)	One Health Plan of Florida	TAMPA: One Health Plan of Florida; ORLAN: One Health Plan of Florida
Preferred Medical Plan (Broward and Miami-Dade counties)	Preferred Medical Plan	SOFLA: Preferred Medical Plan
Total Health Choice (South, central, and eastern Florida)	Total Health Choice	SOFLA: Total Health Choice
UnitedHealthcare of Florida (Most of Florida)	United Healthcare Plan	SOFLA: UnitedHealthcare of Florida; TAMPA: UnitedHealthcare of Florida; ORLAN: UnitedHealthcare of Florida; FTMEY: UnitedHealthcare of Florida
WellCare HMO (South, central, and western Florida)	Well Care HMO	SOFLA: Well Care HMO; TAMPA: Well Care HMO; ORLAN: Well Care HMO; FTMEY: Well Care HMO

Plan	Plan's name as listed in member satisfaction data source	Doctors survey area(s) and how plan's name appeared on survey(s)
	Georgia	
Aetna U.S. Healthcare (Athens, Atlanta, and Augusta areas)	Aetna U.S. Healthcare, Inc. - Georgia	ATLAN: Aetna U.S. Healthcare
BlueCross BlueShield of Georgia (Most of Georgia)	BlueCross BlueShield Healthcare Plan of Georgia, Inc.	ATLAN: BlueChoice (BC/BS of Georgia)
CIGNA HealthCare of Georgia (Northern Georgia)	No data	ATLAN: CIGNA HealthCare of Georgia
Coventry Health Care of Georgia (Atlanta)	No data	ATLAN: Coventry Health Care of GA
Humana Health Plans (HMO) (Atlanta area)	Humana Employers Health of Georgia, Inc. (HMO)	ATLAN: Humana Health Plan of GA
Kaiser Permanente Georgia (HMO) (Atlanta area)	Kaiser Foundation Health Plan of Georgia, Inc. (HMO)	ATLAN: Kaiser Foundation HP of GA
One Health Plan of Georgia (Atlanta and Macon areas)	No data	ATLAN: One Health Plan of Georgia
UnitedHealthcare of Georgia (Most of Georgia)	United HealthCare of Georgia	ATLAN: UnitedHealthcare of Georgia
	Guam	
PacifiCare Asia Pacific (HMO) (Guam)	PacifiCare Asia Pacific (HMO)	No data
	Hawaii	
Health Plan Hawaii (HMO) (Most of HI)	Health Plan Hawaii (HMO)	No data
HMSA (All of Hawaii)	HMSA	No data
Kaiser Permanente Hawaii (HMO) (Most of Hawaii)	Kaiser Foundation Health Plan of Hawaii, Inc. (HMO)	No data
	Idaho	
Group Health Cooperative (HMO) (Northern Idaho)	Group Health Cooperative of Puget Sound (HMO)	SEATT: Group Health Cooperative
Group Health Options (Northern Idaho)	Group Health Options, Inc.	No data
Group Health Options (POS) (Northern Idaho)	Group Health Options, Inc. (POS)	No data
Intermountain Health Care (Southern ID)	IHC	SALTL: IHC Care
	Illinois	
Aetna U.S. Healthcare (Chicago area)	Aetna U.S. Healthcare of Illinois Inc.	CHICA: Aetna U.S. Healthcare of Illinois
Aetna U.S. Healthcare (St. Louis area)	No data	STLOU: Aetna U.S. Healthcare/Prudential
BlueCHOICE (St. Louis area)	HMO Missouri, Inc. d/b/a BlueCHOICE	STLOU: BlueChoice/HMO Missouri
BlueChoice (POS) (Chicago, Rockford, Springfield, St. Louis areas)	BlueChoice (POS)	No data
CIGNA HealthCare of Illinois (Most of IL)	CIGNA HealthCare of Illinois, Inc.	CHICA: CIGNA HealthCare of Illinois
CIGNA HealthCare of St. Louis (St. Louis)	CIGNA HealthCare of St. Louis, Inc.	STLOU: CIGNA HealthCare of St. Louis
Group Health Plan (St. Louis area)	Group Health Plan, Inc.	STLOU: Group Health Plan
Health Alliance (Central and southern IL)	Health Alliance Medical Plans	No data
HealthLink (HMO) (Central and southern Illinois)	HealthLink, Inc. (HMO)	STLOU: HealthLink HMO
HealthLink (POS) (Central and southern Illinois)	HealthLink, Inc. (POS)	STLOU: HealthLink HMO
HMO IL/BlueAdvantage (HMO) (Chi., Peor., Rockford, Sprgf'd, St. L)	HMO Illinois and Blue Advantage HMO (HMO)	CHICA: HMO Illinois
Humana Health Plan–Illinois (HMO) (Chicago area)	Humana Health Plan, Inc. (Illinois) (HMO)	CHICA: Humana Health Plan
John Deere Health Plan (HMO) (Central and northwestern Illinois)	John Deere Health Care, Inc. (HMO)	No data
Medical Associates Health Plans (Jo Daviess County)	Medical Associates Health Plan, Inc. dba Medical Associates Health Plans	No data
Mercy Health Plans (HMO) (St. Louis area)	Mercy Health Plan of Missouri, Inc. (HMO)	STLOU: Mercy Health Plan of Missouri
One Health Plan of Illinois (Chicago area)	No data	CHICA: One Health Plan of Illinois
OSF HealthCare (Northeastern Illinois)	OSF Health Plans, Inc.	No data
PersonalCare (HMO) (East-central IL)	PersonalCare Insurance of IL, Inc. (HMO)	No data
Premier Plus by Mercy Health Plans (HMO) (St. Louis area)	Mercy Health Plans/Premier (HMO)	No data
UNICARE Health Plans of the Midwest (HMO) (Chicago area)	UNICARE Health Plans of the Midwest, Inc. (HMO)	No data
UnitedHealthcare of the Midwest (Southern Illinois)	United HealthCare of the Midwest, Inc. - Combined	STLOU: UnitedHealthcare of the Midwest
	Indiana	
Aetna U.S. Healthcare (Indianapolis area)	Aetna U.S. Healthcare, Inc. - Ohio	CINCI: Aetna U.S. Healthcare; COLUM: Aetna U.S. Healthcare; CLEVE: Aetna U.S. Healthcare; INDIA: Aetna U.S. Healthcare
Aetna U.S. Healthcare (Northwestern IN)	Aetna U.S. Healthcare of Illinois Inc.	CHICA: Aetna U.S. Healthcare of Illinois
Aetna U.S. Healthcare (Southern Indiana)	Aetna USHC Kentucky	No data

Plan	Plan's name as listed in member satisfaction data source	Doctors survey area(s) and how plan's name appeared on survey(s)
Anthem Blue Cross and Blue Shield (Most of Indiana)	Anthem Insurance Companies, Inc. d/b/a Anthem Blue Cross and Blue Shield - Indiana	INDIA: Anthem Health Plan of Indiana
Arnett Health Plans (North-central IN)	Arnett Health Plans	No data
BlueChoice (POS) (Northwestern IN)	BlueChoice (POS)	No data
CIGNA HealthCare of Illinois (Northwestern Indiana)	CIGNA HealthCare of Illinois, Inc.	CHICA: CIGNA HealthCare of Illinois
CIGNA HealthCare of Indiana (Northern and central Indiana)	CIGNA HealthCare of Indiana, Inc	No data
HMO Illinois/BlueAdvantage (HMO) (Northwestern Indiana)	HMO Illinois and Blue Advantage HMO (HMO)	CHICA: HMO Illinois
Humana Health Plan–Illinois (HMO) (Northwestern Indiana)	Humana Health Plan, Inc. (Illinois) (HMO)	CHICA: Humana Health Plan
Humana Health Plans (Southern Indiana)	Humana Health Plan, Inc. (Kentucky)	No data
Humana/ChoiceCare (Southeastern Indiana)	Humana Health Plans of Ohio, Inc. dba ChoiceCare/Humana	CINCI: Humana/ChoiceCare; COLUM: Humana Health Plan of Ohio
M•Plan (HMO) (Northeastern and central Indiana)	M- Plan, Inc. (HMO)	INDIA: M*Plan
PARTNERS National Health Plans of Indiana (Northern Indiana)	PARTNERS National Health Plans of Indiana	No data
UNICARE Health Plans of the Midwest (HMO) (Northwestern Indiana)	UNICARE Health Plans of the Midwest, Inc. (HMO)	No data
UnitedHealthcare of Kentucky (Southern Indiana)	United HealthCare of Kentucky, Ltd.	No data
UnitedHealthcare of Ohio (Dearborn County)	United HealthCare of Ohio, Inc. - Southwest	CINCI: UnitedHealthcare of Ohio
Welborn Health Plans (Southwestern IN)	Welborn HMO	No data
Iowa		
Community Health Plan (Southwestern Iowa)	Community Health Plan	KCITY: Community Health Plan
Coventry Health Care of Iowa (Central IA)	Coventry Health Care of Iowa	No data
Exclusive Healthcare (Western Iowa)	Exclusive Healthcare, Inc. Midwest Region	No data
Health Alliance (Eastern Iowa)	Health Alliance Medical Plans	No data
John Deere Health Plan (HMO) (Central and southeastern Iowa)	John Deere Health Care, Inc. (HMO)	No data
Medical Associates Health Plans (Northeastern Iowa)	Medical Associates Health Plan, Inc. dba Medical Associates Health Plans	No data
Sioux Valley Health Plan (HMO) (Northwestern Iowa)	Sioux Valley Health Plan (HMO)	No data
UnitedHealthcare of the Midlands (Western Iowa)	UnitedHealthcare of the Midlands, Inc.	No data
Wellmark Health Plan of Iowa (Central Iowa)	Wellmark Health Plan of Iowa, Inc.	No data
Kansas		
Aetna U.S. Healthcare (Kansas City area)	U.S. Healthcare, Inc. d/b/a Aetna U.S. Healthcare, a Missouri Corporation (Kansas City)	KCITY: Aetna U.S. Healthcare
Blue Cross Blue Shield of Kansas (HMO) (Most of Kansas)	Blue Cross Blue Shield of Kansas (HMO)	No data
Blue Cross Blue Shield of Kansas (POS) (Most of Kansas)	Blue Cross Blue Shield of Kansas (POS)	No data
BCBS of Kansas City/Blue-Advantage (HMO) (Kansas City area)	Blue Cross and Blue Shield of Kansas City, TriSource Health Care, Inc. & Good Health (HMO)	KCITY: BC/BS of Kansas City
BCBS of Kansas City/Blue-Care (HMO) (Kansas City area)	Blue Cross and Blue Shield of Kansas City, Good Health HMO, Inc. (HMO)	KCITY: BC/BS of Kansas City
CIGNA HealthCare of Kansas/Missouri (Kansas City area)	CIGNA HealthCare of Kansas/Missouri	KCITY: CIGNA HealthCare of KS/MO
Community Health Plan (Northeastern Kansas)	Community Health Plan	KCITY: Community Health Plan
Coventry Health Care of Kansas (Kansas City area)	Coventry Health Care of Kansas, Inc.	KCITY: Coventry Health Care of Kansas
FirstGuard Health Plan (Most or all of KS)	FirstGuard Health Plan, Inc.	KCITY: FirstGuard Health Plan
Humana Health Plans (HMO) (Kansas City area)	Humana Health Plan, Inc./ Humana Kansas City, Inc. (HMO)	KCITY: Humana HMO
Mid America Health (HMO) (Kansas City)	Mid America Health (HMO)	KCITY: HealthNet
Mid America Health (POS) (Kansas City)	Mid America Health (POS)	KCITY: HealthNet
UnitedHealthcare of the Midwest (Eastern Kansas)	UnitedHealthcare of the Midwest, Inc. - Kansas City	KCITY: United Healthcare of the Midwest
Kentucky		
Aetna U.S. Healthcare (Lexington and Louisville areas)	Aetna USHC Kentucky	No data
Aetna U.S. Healthcare (Northern Kentucky)	Aetna U.S. Healthcare, Inc. - Ohio	CINCI: Aetna U.S. Healthcare; COLUM: Aetna U.S. Healthcare; CLEVE: Aetna U.S. Healthcare; INDIA: Aetna U.S. Healthcare

Plan	Plan's name as listed in member satisfaction data source	Doctors survey area(s) and how plan's name appeared on survey(s)
Anthem Blue Cross & Blue Shield (Central, eastern, and northern KY)	Anthem Health Plans of Kentucky, Inc. dba Anthem Blue Cross and Blue Shield	No data
Bluegrass Family Health (Most of KY)	Bluegrass Family Health	No data
CHA Health (Most of Kentucky)	CHA HMO, Inc. d/b/a CHA Health	No data
CIGNA HealthCare Ohio (Northern Kentucky)	CIGNA HealthCare Ohio, Inc.	CINCI: CIGNA HealthCare of Ohio; COLUM: CIGNA HealthCare of Ohio; CLEVE: CIGNA HealthCare of Ohio
Humana Health Plans (Louisville area)	Humana Health Plan, Inc. (Kentucky)	No data
Humana/ChoiceCare (Northern Kentucky)	Humana Health Plans of Ohio, Inc. dba ChoiceCare/Humana	CINCI: Humana/ChoiceCare; COLUM: Humana Health Plan of Ohio
UnitedHealthcare of Kentucky (Most of Kentucky)	United HealthCare of Kentucky, Ltd.	No data
UnitedHealthcare of Ohio (Northern Kentucky)	United HealthCare of Ohio, Inc. - Southwest	CINCI: UnitedHealthcare of Ohio
Louisiana		
Aetna U.S. Healthcare (Southeastern LA)	Aetna U.S. Healthcare	NEWOR: Aetna U.S. Healthcare
CIGNA HealthCare of Louisiana (Southeastern Louisiana)	No data	NEWOR: CIGNA HealthCare of Louisiana
The OATH for Louisiana (All of Louisiana)	No data	NEWOR: The OATH for Louisiana
Ochsner Health Plan (HMO) (Southeastern Louisiana)	Ochsner Health Plan (HMO)	No data
UnitedHealthcare of Louisiana (All or most of Louisiana)	No data	NEWOR: UnitedHealthcare of Louisiana
Maine		
Aetna U.S. Healthcare (All or most of ME)	Aetna U.S. Healthcare Inc. - Maine	No data
Anthem Blue Cross and Blue Shield (All or most of Maine)	Anthem Health Plans of Maine, Inc. d/b/a Anthem Blue Cross and Blue Shield	No data
CIGNA HealthCare of Maine (Most of ME)	CIGNA HealthCare of Maine, Inc.	No data
Harvard Pilgrim Health Care (All or most of Maine)	Harvard Pilgrim Health Care, Inc.	BOSTN: Harvard Pilgrim Health Care
HMO New England (All or most of Maine)	No data	FAIRF: HMO New England; HARTF: HMO New England
Maine Partners Health Plan (Southwestern Maine)	Maine Partners Health Plan	No data
Maryland		
Aetna U.S. Healthcare (Eastern and central Maryland)	Aetna U.S. Healthcare Inc. - Maryland, DC and Virginia	WASDC: Aetna U.S. Healthcare; BALTI: Aetna U.S. Healthcare
AmeriHealth HMO of Delaware (Eastern Maryland)	AmeriHealth HMO, Inc. Delaware	PHILA: AmeriHealth HMO
Capital Care/CareFirst (Washington area)	Capital Care, Inc.	WASDC: CapitalCare; BALTI: CareFirst BlueCross BlueShield
CIGNA HealthCare Mid-Atlantic (Central Maryland)	CIGNA HealthCare Mid-Atlantic, Inc.	WASDC: CIGNA HealthCare Mid-Atlantic; BALTI: CIGNA HealthCare Mid-Atlantic
Coventry Health Care (Most of Maryland)	Coventry Health Care of Delaware, Inc.	PHILA: Conventry Health Care of Delaware; WASDC: Coventry Health Care of Delaware
Delmarva Health Plan (Eastern shore)	Delmarva Health Plan, Inc.	No data
Free State Health Plan (All of Maryland)	Free State Health Plan, Inc.	WASDC: FreeState Health Plan; BALTI: FreeState Health Plan
Kaiser Foundation HP Mid-Atlantic States (HMO) (Central MD)	Kaiser Foundation Health Plan of the Mid-Atlantic States, Inc. (HMO)	WASDC: Kaiser Foundation Health Plan; BALTI: Kaiser Foundation Health Plan
M.D. IPA (All of Maryland)	MD - Individual Practice Association, Inc.	WASDC: M.D. IPA; BALTI: M.D. IPA; NORFO: M.D. IPA
Optimum Choice (All of Maryland)	Optimum Choice, Inc.	WASDC: Optimum Choice; BALTI: Optimum Choice; NORFO: Optimum Choice
Preferred Health Network (Eastern and central Maryland)	The Preferred Health Network	WASDC: PHN-HMO (Preferred Hlth Netwk); BALTI: PHN-HMO
UnitedHealthcare of the Mid-Atlantic (HMO) (All or most of Maryland)	United Healthcare of the Mid-Atlantic (HMO)	WASDC: UnitedHealthcare Mid-Atlantic; BALTI: UnitedHealthcare Mid-Atlantic
Massachusetts		
Aetna U.S. Healthcare (All or most of Massachusetts)	Aetna U.S. Healthcare Inc. - Massachusetts	BOSTN: Aetna U.S. Healthcare; RHODE: Aetna U.S. Healthcare
BlueCHiP (Southeastern Massachusetts)	Coordinated Health Partners, Inc., dba BlueCHiP	BOSTN: Coordinated Hlth Partners/Blue CHiP; RHODE: Coordinated Hlth Partners (Blue CHiP)
BlueCross BlueShield of MA/ HMO Blue (All or most of MA)	Blue Cross and Blue Shield of Massachusetts, Inc.	BOSTN: HMO Blue (BC/BS of MA)
CIGNA HealthCare of Massachusetts (Most of Massachusetts)	CIGNA HealthCare of Massachusetts, Inc.	BOSTN: CIGNA HealthCare of MA
ConnectiCare (Southwestern Massachusetts)	ConnectiCare, Inc.	FAIRF: ConnectiCare; HARTF: ConnectiCare
Fallon Community Health Plan (Eastern and central Massachusetts)	Fallon Community Health Plan	BOSTN: Fallon Community Health Plan
Harvard Pilgrim Health Care (All or most of Massachusetts)	Harvard Pilgrim Health Care, Inc.	BOSTN: Harvard Pilgrim Health Care

Plan	Plan's name as listed in member satisfaction data source	Doctors survey area(s) and how plan's name appeared on survey(s)
Health New England (Western MA)	Health New England, Inc.	No data
HMO New England (All or most of Massachusetts)	No data	FAIRF: HMO New England; HARTF: HMO New England
Neighborhood Health Plan (HMO) (Eastern Massachusetts)	Neighborhood Health Plan, Inc. (HMO)	BOSTN: Neighborhood Health Plan
One Health Plan of Massachusetts (Most of Massachusetts)	No data	BOSTN: One Health Plan of Massachusetts
Tufts Health Plan (HMO) (All or most of Massachusetts)	Tufts Associated Health Maintenance Organization, Inc. dba Tufts Health Plan (HMO)	BOSTN: Tufts Health Plan; RHODE: Tufts Health Plan
Tufts Health Plan (POS) (All or most of Massachusetts)	Total Health Plan, Inc. dba Tufts Health Plan (POS)	BOSTN: Tufts Health Plan; RHODE: Tufts Health Plan
UnitedHealthcare of New England (Southeastern and central MA)	United HealthCare of New England, Inc.	BOSTN: UnitedHealthcare of New England; RHODE: UnitedHealthcare of New England

Michigan

Plan	Plan's name as listed in member satisfaction data source	Doctors survey area(s) and how plan's name appeared on survey(s)
Aetna U.S. Healthcare (Detroit area)	No data	DETRO: Aetna U.S. Healthcare
Blue Care Network of Michigan (HMO) (All or most of Michigan)	Blue Care Network of Michigan (HMO)	DETRO: Blue Care Network of Michigan
Blue Cross Blue Shield of Michigan (POS) (All or most of Michigan)	Blue Cross Blue Shield of Michigan (POS)	No data
Care Choices (HMO) (Central Michigan)	Care Choices HMO (HMO)	DETRO: Care Choices HMO
CIGNA HealthCare of Indiana (Southwestern Michigan)	CIGNA HealthCare of Indiana, Inc	No data
Grand Valley Health Plan (HMO) (Grand Rapids area)	Grand Valley Health Plan, Inc (HMO)	No data
HAP (HMO) (Southeastern Michigan)	Health Alliance Plan of Michigan (HMO)	DETRO: HAP
HealthPlus of Michigan (Central MI)	HealthPlus of Michigan	DETRO: HealthPlus of Michigan
M-CARE (HMO) (Southeastern Michigan)	M-CARE, Inc. (HMO)	DETRO: M-CARE
OmniCare Health Plan (HMO) (Southeastern Michigan)	OmniCare Health Plan (HMO)	DETRO: OmniCare Heath Plan
OmniCare Health Plan (POS) (Southeastern Michigan)	OmniCare Health Plan (POS)	DETRO: OmniCare Heath Plan
Paramount Health Care (HMO) (Southeastern Michigan)	Paramount Care, Inc. dba Paramount Health Care (HMO)	No data
Physicians Health Plan of Mid-Michigan (Central Michigan)	Physicians Health Plan of Mid-Michigan	No data
Physicians Health Plan of South Michigan (South-central Michigan)	Physicians Health Plan of South Michigan	No data
Physicians Health Plan of Southwest Michigan (Southwestern MI)	Physicians Health Plan of Southwest MI, Inc.	No data
Priority Health (HMO) (Most of western Michigan)	Priority Health (HMO)	No data
Total Health Care (Southeastern MI)	No data	DETRO: Total Health Care
Ultimed HMO of Michigan (Detroit area)	No data	DETRO: Ultimed HMO of Michigan
The Wellness Plan (HMO) (Southeastern Michigan)	The Wellness Plan (HMO)	DETRO: The Wellness Plan

Minnesota

Plan	Plan's name as listed in member satisfaction data source	Doctors survey area(s) and how plan's name appeared on survey(s)
Blue Plus (All or most of Minnesota)	Blue Plus (HMO Minnesota d/b/a Blue Plus)	TWINC: Blue Plus
HealthPartners Classic (Twin Cities area)	HealthPartners Classic	TWINC: HealthPartners
Medica (Most of Minnesota)	Medica Health Plans	TWINC: Medica
PreferredOne (Most of Minnesota)	No data	TWINC: PreferredOne
Sioux Valley Health Plan (HMO) (Southwestern Minnesota)	Sioux Valley Health Plan (HMO)	No data
Sioux Valley Health Plan of Minnesota (HMO) (Southwestern MN)	Sioux Valley Health Plan of Minnesota (HMO)	No data

Mississippi

Plan	Plan's name as listed in member satisfaction data source	Doctors survey area(s) and how plan's name appeared on survey(s)
Aetna U.S. Healthcare (Northwestern Mississippi)	Prudential HealthCare Plan, Inc., A Member Company of Aetna U.S. Healthcare - Memphis	No data
CIGNA HealthCare of Louisiana (Pearl River and Hancock counties)	No data	NEWOR: CIGNA HealthCare of Louisiana

Missouri

Plan	Plan's name as listed in member satisfaction data source	Doctors survey area(s) and how plan's name appeared on survey(s)
Aetna U.S. Healthcare (Kansas City area)	U.S. Healthcare, Inc. d/b/a Aetna U.S. Healthcare, a Missouri Corporation (Kansas City)	KCITY: Aetna U.S. Healthcare
Aetna U.S. Healthcare (St. Louis area)	No data	STLOU: Aetna U.S. Healthcare/Prudential
BCBS of Kansas City/Blue-Advantage (HMO) (Kansas City area)	Blue Cross and Blue Shield of Kansas City, TriSource Health Care, Inc. & Good Health	KCITY: BC/BS of Kansas City
BCBS of Kansas City/Blue-Care (HMO) (Kansas City area)	Blue Cross and Blue Shield of Kansas City, Good Health HMO, Inc. (HMO)	KCITY: BC/BS of Kansas City
BlueCHOICE (Eastern and southern MO)	HMO Missouri, Inc. d/b/a BlueCHOICE	STLOU: BlueChoice/HMO Missouri
CIGNA HealthCare of Kansas/Missouri (Kansas City area)	CIGNA HealthCare of Kansas/Missouri	KCITY: CIGNA HealthCare of KS/MO
CIGNA HealthCare of St. Louis (St. Louis)	CIGNA HealthCare of St. Louis, Inc.	STLOU: CIGNA HealthCare of St. Louis
Community Health Plan (Northwestern Missouri)	Community Health Plan	KCITY: Community Health Plan
Coventry Health Care of Kansas (Kansas City area)	Coventry Health Care of Kansas, Inc.	KCITY: Coventry Health Care of Kansas
Cox HealthPlans (Southwestern Missouri)	Cox Health Systems HMO, Inc.	No data
FirstGuard Health Plan (Kansas City area)	FirstGuard Health Plan, Inc.	KCITY: FirstGuard Health Plan
Group Health Plan (St. Louis area)	Group Health Plan, Inc.	STLOU: Group Health Plan
HealthLink (HMO) (Northeastern, east-central, and southwestern MO)	HealthLink, Inc. (HMO)	STLOU: HealthLink HMO
HealthLink (POS) (Northeastern, east-central, and southwestern MO)	HealthLink, Inc. (POS)	STLOU: HealthLink HMO
Humana Health Plans (Kansas City area)	Humana Health Plan, Inc./ Humana Kansas City, Inc. (HMO)	KCITY: Humana HMO
Mercy Health Plans (HMO) (Eastern and central Missouri)	Mercy Health Plan of Missouri, Inc. (HMO)	STLOU: Mercy Health Plan of Missouri
Mid America Health (HMO) (Kansas City)	Mid America Health (HMO)	KCITY: HealthNet
Mid America Health (POS) (Kansas City)	Mid America Health (POS)	KCITY: HealthNet
Premier Health Plans (HMO) (Southwestern Missouri)	Premier Health Plans (Mercy Health Plans of MO/Southwest MO) (HMO)	No data
Premier Plus by Mercy Health Plans (HMO) (Eastern Missouri)	Mercy Health Plans/Premier (HMO)	No data
UnitedHealthcare of the Midwest (Most of eastern Missouri)	United HealthCare of the Midwest, Inc. - Combined	STLOU: UnitedHealthcare of the Midwest
UnitedHealthcare of the Midwest (Most of western Missouri)	UnitedHealthcare of the Midwest, Inc. - Kansas City	KCITY: United Healthcare of the Midwest

Nebraska

Plan	Plan's name as listed in member satisfaction data source	Doctors survey area(s) and how plan's name appeared on survey(s)
Exclusive Healthcare (Eastern Nebraska)	Exclusive Healthcare, Inc. Midwest	No data
Sioux Valley Health Plan (HMO) (Northeastern Nebraska)	Sioux Valley Health Plan (HMO)	No data
UnitedHealthcare of the Midlands (Eastern Nebraska)	UnitedHealthcare of the Midlands, Inc.	No data

Nevada

Plan	Plan's name as listed in member satisfaction data source	Doctors survey area(s) and how plan's name appeared on survey(s)
Aetna U.S. Healthcare (Southern Nevada)	Aetna U.S. Healthcare, Inc. - Nevada	VEGAS: Aetna U.S. Healthcare
Health Plan of Nevada (Southern and western Nevada)	Health Plan of Nevada, Inc.	VEGAS: Health Plan of Nevada
HMO Nevada (All or most of Nevada)	No data	VEGAS: HMO Nevada
NevadaCare (Las Vegas area)	No data	VEGAS: NevadaCare
PacifiCare of Nevada (HMO) (Southern and western Nevada)	PacifiCare of Nevada, Inc. (HMO)	VEGAS: PacifiCare of Nevada

New Hampshire

Plan	Plan's name as listed in member satisfaction data source	Doctors survey area(s) and how plan's name appeared on survey(s)
Anthem Blue Cross and Blue Shield (All or most of New Hampshire)	Anthem Health Plans of New Hampshire, Inc. d/b/a/ Anthem Blue Cross and Blue Shield	No data
BlueCross BlueShield of MA/HMO Blue (Southeastern NH)	Blue Cross and Blue Shield of Massachusetts, Inc.	BOSTN: HMO Blue (BC/BS of MA)
CIGNA HealthCare of New Hampshire (All of New Hampshire)	CIGNA HealthCare of New Hampshire, Inc.	No data
Harvard Pilgrim Health Care of New England (Most of NH)	Harvard Pilgrim Health Care of New England (NH/VT)	No data
HMO New England (All or most of New Hampshire)	No data	FAIRF: HMO New England; HARTF: HMO New England
Tufts Health Plan (HMO) (Southern New Hampshire)	Tufts Associated Health Maintenance Organization, Inc. dba Tufts Health Plan (HMO)	BOSTN: Tufts Health Plan; RHODE: Tufts Health Plan
Tufts Health Plan (POS) (Southern New Hampshire)	Total Health Plan, Inc. dba Tufts Health Plan (POS)	BOSTN: Tufts Health Plan; RHODE: Tufts Health Plan

New Jersey

Plan	Plan's name as listed in member satisfaction data source	Doctors survey area(s) and how plan's name appeared on survey(s)
Aetna U.S. Healthcare (Northern NJ)	Aetna U.S. Healthcare - Northern NJ	JERSE: Aetna U.S. Healthcare
Aetna U.S. Healthcare (Southern NJ)	Aetna U.S. Healthcare Southern NJ	PHILA: Aetna U.S. Healthcare (NJ)
AmeriHealth HMO of New Jersey (All of New Jersey)	AmeriHealth HMO Inc. - New Jersey	NYORK: AmeriHealth Health Plan; JERSE: AmeriHealth HMO; PHILA: AmeriHealth HMO
CIGNA HealthCare of New Jersey (All of New Jersey)	CIGNA Health Care of NJ	JERSE: CIGNA HealthCare of New Jersey; PHILA: CIGNA HealthCare of New Jersey
Coventry Health Care (Southwestern New Jersey)	Coventry Health Care of Delaware, Inc.	PHILA: Conventry Health Care of Delaware; WASDC: Coventry Health Care of Delaware
Health Net of the Northeast (All of New Jersey)	Health Net, Inc.	NYORK: Physicians Health Svcs of NY; JERSE: Health Net (formerly PHS); PHILA: Physicians Health Services of NJ
Horizon HMO (HMO) (All of New Jersey)	Horizon Healthcare of New Jersey, Inc. d/b/a Horizon HMO (HMO)	PHILA: Horizon HMO; JERSE: Horizon HMO (BC/BS of NJ)
Keystone Health Plan East (All or most of New Jersey)	Keystone Health Plan East, Inc.	PHILA: Keystone Health Plan East; JERSE: Keystone Health Plan East
One Health Plan (All or most of NJ)	One Health Plan of New Jersey	JERSE: One Health Plan of New Jersey

Plan	Plan's name as listed in member satisfaction data source	Doctors survey area(s) and how plan's name appeared on survey(s)
Oxford Health Plans (All or most of New Jersey)	Oxford Health Plans - New Jersey	JERSE: Oxford Health Plans of NJ; PHILA: Oxford Health Plans of NJ
UnitedHealthcare of New Jersey (All or most of New Jersey)	United Healthcare of New Jersey, Inc.	JERSE: UnitedHealthcare of New Jersey; PHILA: United HealthCare of New Jersey
University Health Plans (All of New Jersey)	No data	JERSE: University Health Plans; PHILA: University Health Plans
WellChoice HMO of New Jersey (Northern New Jersey)	WellChoice	No data

New Mexico

Plan	Plan's name as listed in member satisfaction data source	Doctors survey area(s) and how plan's name appeared on survey(s)
Blue Cross and Blue Shield of NM (POS) (All or most of NM)	New Mexico Blue Cross and Blue Shield Inc. (POS)	No data
Cimarron Health Plan (All or most of NM)	Cimarron Health Plan	No data
HMO New Mexico (HMO) (All or most of New Mexico)	HMO New Mexico, Inc. subsidiary of New Mexico Blue Cross and Blue Shield (HMO)	No data
Lovelace Health Systems (All or most of New Mexico)	Lovelace Health Systems, Inc.	No data
Presbyterian Health Plan (All or most of New Mexico)	Presbyterian Health Plan, Inc.	No data

New York

Plan	Plan's name as listed in member satisfaction data source	Doctors survey area(s) and how plan's name appeared on survey(s)
Aetna U.S. Healthcare (NYC, Long Island, Downstate NY, Bing., Syr.)	U.S. Healthcare, Inc. (New York) dba Aetna U.S. Healthcare	NYORK: Aetna U.S. Healthcare
Atlantis Health Plan (NYC, Long Island, Westchester & Rockland cos)	No data	NYORK: Atlantis Health Plan
BlueCross Blue Shield of Western NY/ Community Blue (Western NY)	Community Blue/Blue Cross and Blue Shield of Western New York	BUFFA: Community Blue (BCBS)
BlueShield of Northeastern New York (Northeastern New York)	Blue Shield of Northeastern New York	No data
Capital District Physicians' Health Plan (Eastern Upstate New York)	C.D.P.H.P.	No data
CIGNA HealthCare of NY (NYC, Long Island, and Downstate NY)	CIGNA Health Care of NY	NYORK: CIGNA HealthCare of New York
Empire BlueCross BlueShield (HMO) (Eastern and Downstate NY)	Empire Blue Cross Blue Shield (HMO)	NYORK: Empire BC/BS Healthnet
Excellus Health Plan/Blue Choice (Rochester area)	Excellus Health Plan, Inc. - Blue Choice - Rochester Area Division	ROCHE: Blue Choice
GHI HMO Select (HMO) (NYC and eastern New York)	GHI HMO Select (HMO)	NYORK: GHI HMO Select
Health Net of the Northeast (NYC, Long Island, and Downstate NY)	Health Net, Inc.	NYORK: Physicians Health Svcs of NY; JERSE: Health Net (formerly PHS); PHILA: Physicians Health Services of NJ
Healthfirst New York (New York City)	No data	NYORK: Healthfirst New York
HIP Health Plan (NYC, Long Island, and Downstate New York)	HIP Health Plan of New York	NYORK: HIP Health Plan of New York
HMO Blue (HMO) (Rome, Utica, and Watertown areas)	Excellus Health Plan, Inc. dba HMO Blue (HMO)	No data
HMO-CNY (HMO) (Central New York)	Excellus Health Plan Inc., d/b/a HMO-CNY (HMO)	No data
Independent Health (HMO) (Western New York)	Independent Health (HMO)	BUFFA: Independent Health
MagnaHealth (NYC, Long Island, and Westchester County)	No data	NYORK: MagnaHealth
MDNY Healthcare (Long Island)	No data	NYORK: MDNY Healthcare
MVP Health Care (HMO) (Central and eastern Upstate NY & So. Tier)	MVP Health Plan (HMO)	No data
Oxford Health Plans (NYC, Long Island, and Downstate New York)	Oxford Health Plans - New York	NYORK: Oxford Health Plans of New York
Preferred Care (Rochester area)	Rochester Area Health Maintenance Organization d.b.a. Preferred Care	ROCHE: Preferred Care
UnitedHealthcare of NY (NYC, Long Island, and Downstate NY)	United HealthCare of New York, Inc.	NYORK: UnitedHealthcare of New York; FAIRF: UnitedHealthcare
UnitedHealthcare of Upstate New York (Upstate New York)	United HealthCare of Upstate New York, Inc. / United HealthCare Insurance Co. NY	No data
Univera Healthcare Central New York (Syracuse area)	Univera Healthcare - CNY, Inc. (formerly HSMC) dba Prepaid Health Plan	No data
Univera Healthcare Western New York (Western New York)	Univera Healthcare - Western New York	BUFFA: Univera Healthcare
Vytra Health Plans (Long Island and Queens)	Vytra Health Plans Long Island Inc.	NYORK: Vytra Health Plans

North Carolina

Plan	Plan's name as listed in member satisfaction data source	Doctors survey area(s) and how plan's name appeared on survey(s)
Aetna U.S. Healthcare (Charlotte and Triangle areas)	Aetna U.S. Healthcare, Inc. - Carolinas	CHARL: Aetna U.S. Healthcare; TRIAN: Aetna U.S. Healthcare
BlueCross BlueShield of NC/Personal Care (All or most of NC)	Blue Cross and Blue Shield of North Carolina and Personal Care Plan of North Carolina, Inc.	CHARL: Personal Care Plan (BC/BS of NC); WSALM: BCBS of NC Personal Care Plan; TRIAN: BCBS of NC Personal Care Plan
CIGNA HealthCare of North Carolina (All of North Carolina)	CIGNA HealthCare of North Carolina, Inc.	CHARL: CIGNA HealthCare of NC; WSALM: CIGNA HealthCare of NC; TRIAN: CIGNA HealthCare of NC

Plan	Plan's name as listed in member satisfaction data source	Doctors survey area(s) and how plan's name appeared on survey(s)
Coventry Health Care Carolinas (Charlotte area)	Coventry Health Care of the Carolina	CHARL: Coventry Health Care Carolinas
Doctors Health Plan (Charlotte, Fayetteville, Triangle, Wilmington)	Doctors Health Plan	CHARL: Doctors Health Plan; WSALM: Doctors Health Plan; TRIAN: Doctors Health Plan
One Health Plan (HMO) (Charlotte, Greensboro, Triangle, Winst.-Sal.)	One Health Plan of North Carolina, Inc (HMO)	No data
Optimum Choice of the Carolinas (Char., Greens., Tri., Winst.-Sal.)	Optimum Choice of the Carolinas, Inc	CHARL: Optimim Choice of the Carolinas; WSALM: Optimum Choice of the Carolinas; TRIAN: Optimum Choice of the Carolinas
PARTNERS National Health Plan of NC (All or most of NC)	PARTNERS National Health Plan of North Carolina	CHARL: PARTNERS Nat'l HPs of NC; WSALM: PARTNERS Health Plans; TRIAN: PARTNERS Health Plans
UnitedHealthcare of North Carolina (Most of North Carolina)	UnitedHealthcare of North Carolina, Inc.	CHARL: UnitedHealthcare of NC; WSALM: United Healthcare of NC; TRIAN: UnitedHealthcare of NC
WellPath Select (Most of North Carolina)	WellPath Select, Inc.	CHARL: WellPath Select; WSALM: WellPath Select; TRIAN: WellPath Select

Ohio

Plan	Plan's name as listed in member satisfaction data source	Doctors survey area(s) and how plan's name appeared on survey(s)
Aetna U.S. Healthcare (Most of Ohio)	Aetna U.S. Healthcare, Inc. - Ohio	CINCI: Aetna U.S. Healthcare; COLUM: Aetna U.S. Healthcare; CLEVE: Aetna U.S. Healthcare; INDIA: Aetna U.S. Healthcare
Anthem Blue Cross and Blue Shield (Most of Ohio)	Community Insurance Company dba Anthem Blue Cross and Blue Shield - Ohio	CINCI: Anthem BC/BS; COLUM: Anthem BC/BS; CLEVE: Anthem BCBS-Anthem HMO
AultCare (HMO) (Canton area)	AultCare HMO (HMO)	No data
CIGNA HealthCare Ohio (Most of Ohio)	CIGNA HealthCare Ohio, Inc.	CINCI: CIGNA HealthCare of Ohio; COLUM: CIGNA HealthCare of Ohio; CLEVE: CIGNA HealthCare of Ohio
Family Health Plan (Northwestern Ohio)	Family Health Plan, Inc.	No data
HAP (HMO) (Northwestern Ohio)	Health Alliance Plan of Michigan (HMO)	DETRO: HAP
The Health Plan of the Upper Ohio Valley (HMO) (Southeastern Ohio)	The Health Plan of the Upper Ohio Valley, Inc. (HMO)	No data
HealthAmerica (HMO) (Eastern Ohio)	HealthAmerica Pennsylvania, Inc. (HMO)	PITTS: HealthAmerica of Pennsylvania
HealthAmerica (POS) (Eastern Ohio)	HealthAmerica Pennsylvania, Inc. (POS)	PITTS: HealthAmerica of Pennsylvania
HMO Health Ohio (All of Ohio)	HMO Health Ohio	CINCI: HMO Health Ohio; COLUM: HMO Health Ohio; CLEVE: HMO Health Ohio
HomeTown Health Network (HMO) (Eastern Ohio)	HomeTown Health Network (HMO)	No data
Humana/ChoiceCare (Southern and central Ohio)	Humana Health Plans of Ohio, Inc. dba ChoiceCare/Humana	CINCI: Humana/ChoiceCare; COLUM: Humana Health Plan of Ohio
Kaiser Permanente Ohio (HMO) (Akron, Canton, and Cleveland areas)	Kaiser Foundation Health Plan of Ohio (HMO)	CLEVE: Kaiser Foundation HP of Ohio
Nationwide Health Plans (All of Ohio)	No data	CLEVE: Nationwide Health Plans; CINCI: Nationwide Health Plans; COLUM: Nationwide Health Plans
One Health Plan of Ohio (Parts of Ohio)	No data	CLEVE: One Health Plan of Ohio; CINCI: One Health Plan of Ohio; COLUM: One Health Plan of Ohio
Paramount Health Care (HMO) (Northwestern Ohio)	Paramount Care, Inc. dba Paramount Health Care (HMO)	No data
QualChoice (Northeastern Ohio)	No data	CLEVE: QualChoice Health Plan
SummaCare (Northeastern Ohio)	SummaCare, Inc.	CLEVE: SummaCare Health Plan
SuperMed HMO (Northeastern Ohio)	SuperMed HMO	CLEVE: SuperMed HMO
UnitedHealthcare of Ohio (Central and southeastern Ohio)	United HealthCare of Ohio, Inc. - Columbus	COLUM: United Healthcare of Ohio
UnitedHealthcare of Ohio (Northern Ohio)	United HealthCare of Ohio, Inc. - Northern Ohio Market	CLEVE: UnitedHealthcare of Ohio
UnitedHealthcare of Ohio (Southwestern Ohio)	United HealthCare of Ohio, Inc. - Southwest	CINCI: UnitedHealthcare of Ohio

Oklahoma

Plan	Plan's name as listed in member satisfaction data source	Doctors survey area(s) and how plan's name appeared on survey(s)
PacifiCare of Oklahoma (HMO) (Oklahoma City and Tulsa areas)	PacifiCare of Oklahoma, Inc. (HMO)	No data

Oregon

Plan	Plan's name as listed in member satisfaction data source	Doctors survey area(s) and how plan's name appeared on survey(s)
Health Net Health Plan of Oregon (Most of western Oregon)	No data	PORTL: Health Net Health Plan of Oregon
Kaiser Permanente Northwest (HMO) (Corvallis, Portland, Salem)	Kaiser Foundation Health Plan of the Northwest, Inc. (HMO)	PORTL: Kaiser Permanente Northwest
PacifiCare of Oregon (HMO) (Corvallis, Portland, and Salem areas)	PacifiCare of Oregon, Inc. (HMO)	PORTL: PacifiCare of Oregon
Providence Health Plans (Corvallis, Eugene, Portland, Salem areas)	Providence Health Plans - Oregon	PORTL: Providence Health Plan
Regence HMO Oregon (Eastern Oregon)	Regence HMO Oregon	PORTL: RegenceHMO (BCBS of Oregon)

Plan	Plan's name as listed in member satisfaction data source	Doctors survey area(s) and how plan's name appeared on survey(s)
Pennsylvania		
Aetna U.S. Healthcare (HMO) (Southeastern Pennsylvania)	Aetna U.S. Healthcare, Inc. Southeastern Pennsylvania/Harrisburg (HMO)	PHILA: Aetna U.S. Healthcare (PA & DE)
Aetna U.S. Healthcare (POS) (Southeastern Pennsylvania)	Aetna U.S. Healthcare, Inc. Southeastern Pennsylvania/Harrisburg (POS)	PHILA: Aetna U.S. Healthcare (PA & DE)
Aetna U.S. Healthcare (HMO) (Western Pennsylvania)	Aetna U.S. Healthcare, Inc. - Pittsburgh (HMO)	PITTS: Aetna U.S. Healthcare
Aetna U.S. Healthcare (POS) (Western Pennsylvania)	Aetna U.S. Healthcare, Inc. - Pittsburgh (POS)	PITTS: Aetna U.S. Healthcare
AmeriHealth HMO of New Jersey (Southeastern Pennsylvania)	AmeriHealth HMO Inc. - New Jersey	NYORK: AmeriHealth Health Plan; JERSE: AmeriHealth HMO; PHILA: AmeriHealth HMO
CIGNA HealthCare of Pennsylvania (Southeastern Pennsylvania)	CIGNA HealthCare of Pennsylvania, Inc.	PHILA: CIGNA HealthCare of Pennsylvania
Coventry Health Care (Southeastern Pennsylvania)	Coventry Health Care of Delaware, Inc.	PHILA: Coventry Health Care of Delaware; WASDC: Coventry Health Care of Delaware
First Priority Health (Northeastern Pennsylvania)	HMO of Northeastern Pennsylvania, Inc. d/b/a First Priority Health	No data
Geisinger Health Plan (Central and northeastern Pennsylvania)	Geisinger Health Plan	No data
Health Net of the Northeast (SE PA, Scranton/Wilkes-Barre area)	PHS Health Plans (QualMed Plans for Hlth)	PHILA: QualMed Plans for Health
HealthAmerica (HMO) (Central and western Pennsylvania)	HealthAmerica Pennsylvania, Inc. (HMO)	PITTS: HealthAmerica of Pennsylvania
HealthAmerica (POS) (Central and western Pennsylvania)	HealthAmerica Pennsylvania, Inc. (POS)	PITTS: HealthAmerica of Pennsylvania
HealthGuard (Harrisburg, Lancaster, Reading, and York areas)	HealthGuard of Lancaster, Inc.	No data
Keystone Health Plan Central (HMO) (Central Pennsylvania)	Keystone Health Plan Central (HMO)	No data
Keystone Health Plan East (Eastern Pennsylvania)	Keystone Health Plan East, Inc.	PHILA: Keystone Health Plan East; JERSE: Keystone Health Plan East
Keystone Health Plan West (Western PA)	Keystone Health Plan West, Inc.	PITTS: Keystone Health Plan West
NewAlliance Health Plan (Northwestern Pennsylvania)	NewAlliance Health Plan	No data
UPMC Health Plan (Western PA)	UPMC Health Plan, Inc.	PITTS: UPMC Health Plan
Puerto Rico		
Triple-S (HMO) (All of Puerto Rico)	Triple-S (HMO)	No data
Rhode Island		
Aetna U.S. Healthcare (All or most of Rhode Island)	Aetna U.S. Healthcare Inc. - Massachusetts	BOSTN: Aetna U.S. Healthcare; RHODE: Aetna U.S. Healthcare
BlueCHiP (All of Rhode Island)	Coordinated Health Partners, Inc., dba BlueCHiP	BOSTN: Coordinated Hlth Partners/Blue CHiP; RHODE: Coordinated Hlth Partners (Blue CHiP)
BlueCross BlueShield of MA/ HMO Blue (All or most of RI)	Blue Cross and Blue Shield of Massachusetts, Inc.	BOSTN: HMO Blue (BC/BS of MA)
HMO New England (All or most of Rhode Island)	No data	FAIRF: HMO New England; HARTF: HMO New England
Tufts Health Plan (HMO) (All or most of Rhode Island)	Tufts Associated Health Maintenance Organization, Inc. dba Tufts Health Plan (HMO)	BOSTN: Tufts Health Plan; RHODE: Tufts Health Plan
Tufts Health Plan (POS) (All or most of Rhode Island)	Total Health Plan, Inc. dba Tufts Health Plan (POS)	BOSTN: Tufts Health Plan; RHODE: Tufts Health Plan
UnitedHealthcare of New England (All of Rhode Island)	United HealthCare of New England, Inc.	BOSTN: UnitedHealthcare of New England; RHODE: UnitedHealthcare of New England
South Carolina		
Aetna U.S. Healthcare (B'fort, Charleston, Clmbia, Rock Hill, Spart.)	Aetna U.S. Healthcare, Inc. - Carolinas	CHARL: Aetna U.S. Healthcare; TRIAN: Aetna U.S. Healthcare
Carolina Care Plan (All or most of SC)	Physicians Health Plan, Inc. - SC	No data
CIGNA HealthCare of South Carolina (All of South Carolina)	CIGNA HealthCare of South Carolina, Inc.	No data
Companion HealthCare (All or most of SC)	Companion HealthCare	No data
Coventry Health Care Carolinas (Union and York counties)	Coventry Health Care of the Carolina	CHARL: Coventry Health Care Carolinas
Doctors Health Plan (York County)	Doctors Health Plan	CHARL: Doctors Health Plan; WSALM: Doctors Health Plan; TRIAN: Doctors Health Plan
One Health Plan (HMO) (York County)	One Health Plan of NC, Inc (HMO)	No data
PARTNERS Nat'l HP of NC (Columbia, Grnvlle, Rock Hill, Spartan.)	PARTNERS National Health Plan of North Carolina	CHARL: PARTNERS Nat'l HPs of NC; WSALM: PARTNERS Health Plans; TRIAN: PARTNERS Health Plans
WellPath Select (Anderson, Greenville, Rock Hill, Spartanburg)	WellPath Select, Inc.	CHARL: WellPath Select; WSALM: WellPath Select; TRIAN: WellPath Select

Plan	Plan's name as listed in member satisfaction data source	Doctors survey area(s) and how plan's name appeared on survey(s)
South Dakota		
Exclusive Healthcare (Union County)	Exclusive Healthcare, Inc. Midwest Region	No data
Sioux Valley Health Plan (HMO) (Most of South Dakota)	Sioux Valley Health Plan (HMO)	No data
Tennessee		
Aetna U.S. Healthcare (Central TN)	Aetna U.S. Healthcare, Inc. - Tennessee	NASHV: Aetna U.S. Healthcare
Aetna U.S. Healthcare (Memphis area)	Prudential HealthCare Plan, Inc., A Member Company of Aetna U.S. Healthcare - Memphis	No data
CIGNA HealthCare of Tennessee (Most of Tennessee)	CIGNA HealthCare of Tennessee, Inc.	NASHV: CIGNA HealthCare of Tennessee
HealthSpring (Nashville area)	No data	NASHV: Health Net HMO
HMO Blue (All or most of Tennessee)	Tennessee Health Care Network, Inc.	NASHV: HMO Blue
John Deere Health Plan (HMO) (Eastern Tennessee)	John Deere Health Care, Inc. (HMO)	No data
One Health Plan of Tennessee (Memphis and Nashville areas)	No data	NASHV: One Health Plan of Tennessee
UnitedHealthcare of Tennessee (Most of Tennessee)	United HealthCare of Tennessee, Inc.	NASHV: UnitedHealthcare of Tennessee
Texas		
Aetna U.S. Healthcare (Austin, Corpus Ch., El Paso, Hou., San Ant.)	Aetna U.S. Healthcare Inc. - Houston	AUSTN: Aetna U.S. Healthcare; HOUST: Aetna U.S. Healthcare; SANAN: Aetna U.S. Healthcare
Aetna U.S. Healthcare (Dallas-Ft. Worth)	Aetna U.S. Healthcare of North TX, Inc.	DALLA: Aetna U.S. Healthcare
AmCare Health Plans (Most of Texas)	AmCare Health Plans of Texas	DALLA: AmCare Health Plans of Texas; HOUST: AmCare Health Plans of Texas; SANAN: AmCare Health Plans of Texas; AUSTN: AmCare Health Plans of Texas
Amil International (HMO) (Austin area)	Amil International (Texas) Inc. (HMO)	No data
CIGNA HealthCare of North Texas (Northern Texas)	CIGNA HealthCare of Texas, Inc.	DALLA: CIGNA HealthCare of North Texas
CIGNA HealthCare of South Texas (Southern Texas)	CIGNA HealthCare of Texas, Inc., South Texas Division	HOUST: CIGNA HealthCare of Texas
Community First Health Plans (HMO) (San Antonio area)	Community First Health Plans, Inc. (HMO)	SANAN: Community First Health Plans
FIRSTCARE (HMO) (Abilene area)	SHA, LLC dba FIRSTCARE (HMO)	No data
FIRSTCARE (HMO) (Amarillo area)	SHA, LLC dba FIRSTCARE (HMO)	No data
FIRSTCARE (HMO) (Lubbock area)	SHA, LLC dba FIRSTCARE (HMO)	No data
FIRSTCARE (HMO) (Waco area)	SHA, LLC dba FIRSTCARE (HMO)	No data
Heritage Health Plan (Northeastern Texas)	Health Plan of Texas, Inc. dba Heritage Health Plan	No data
HMO Blue, Central/South TX (HMO) (Most of southern and central TX)	HMO Blue, Central/South Texas (HMO)	AUSTN: HMO Blue, Central Texas; SANAN: HMO Blue, Central Texas
HMO Blue, El Paso (HMO) (El Paso area)	HMO Blue, El Paso (HMO)	No data
HMO Blue, Northeast Texas (HMO) (Dallas-Ft. Worth area)	HMO Blue, Northeast Texas (HMO)	DALLA: HMO Blue, Northeast Texas
HMO Blue, Southeast Texas (HMO) (Houston area)	HMO Blue, Southeast Texas (HMO)	HOUST: HMO Blue, Southeast Texas
HMO Blue, Southwest Texas (HMO) (Abilene and San Angelo areas)	HMO Blue, Southwest Texas (HMO)	No data
HMO Blue, Southwest Texas (HMO) (Midland area)	HMO Blue, Southwest Texas (HMO)	No data
HMO Blue Texas (Austin area)	HMO Blue Texas	AUSTN: HMO Blue Texas
HMO Blue Texas (Beaumont and Lufkin)	HMO Blue Texas	No data
HMO Blue Texas (Dallas-Ft. Worth area)	Southwest Texas HMO, Inc. dba HMO Blue Texas	No data
HMO Blue Texas (Corpus Christi area)	HMO Blue Texas	No data
HMO Blue Texas (Houston area)	HMO Blue Texas	HOUST: HMO Blue Texas
HMO Blue Texas (San Antonio area)	HMO Blue Texas	SANAN: HMO Blue Texas
HMO Blue, West Texas (HMO) (Texas Panhandle)	West Texas Health Plans, L.C. (HMO)	No data
Humana Health Plan of Texas (HMO) (Austin area)	Humana Health Plan of Texas, Inc. (HMO)	AUSTN: Humana Health Plan of Texas
Humana Health Plan of Texas (HMO) (Corpus Christi area)	Humana Health Plan of Texas, Inc. (HMO)	No data
Humana Health Plan of Texas (HMO) (Houston area)	Humana Health Plan of Texas, Inc. (HMO)	HOUST: Humana Health Plan of Texas
Humana Health Plan of Texas (HMO) (San Antonio area)	Humana Health Plan of Texas, Inc. (HMO)	SANAN: Humana Health Plan of Texas
Mercy Health Plans (HMO) (Laredo area)	Mercy Health Plan of Missouri, Inc. (Texas) (HMO)	No data
MethodistCare (HMO) (Southeastern Texas)	MethodistCare, Inc. dba MethodistCare (HMO)	HOUST: MethodistCare
MetroWest Health Plan (Dallas-Ft. Worth)	No data	DALLA: MetroWest Health Plan

Plan	Plan's name as listed in member satisfaction data source	Doctors survey area(s) and how plan's name appeared on survey(s)
One Health Plan of Texas (HMO) (Central and southern Texas)	One Health Plan of Texas, Inc. (HMO)	AUSTN: One Health Plan of Texas; SANAN: One Health Plan of Texas
One Health Plan of Texas (HMO) (Dallas-Ft. Worth area)	One Health Plan of Texas, Inc. (HMO)	DALLA: One Health Plan of Texas
One Health Plan of Texas (HMO) (Houston area)	One Health Plan of Texas, Inc. (HMO)	HOUST: One Health Plan of Texas
PacifiCare of Texas (HMO) (Dallas-Ft. Worth area)	PacifiCare of Texas, Inc. (HMO)	DALLA: PacifiCare of Texas
PacifiCare of Texas (HMO) (Houston)	PacifiCare of Texas, Inc. (HMO)	HOUST: PacifiCare of Texas
PacifiCare of Texas (HMO) (San Antonio area)	PacifiCare of Texas, Inc. (HMO)	SANAN: PacifiCare of Texas; AUSTN: PacifiCare of Texas
Parkland Community Health Plan (HMO) (Dallas area)	Parkland Community Health Plan (HMO)	No data
Scott & White Health Plan (HMO) (Austin and Waco areas)	Scott and White Health Plan (HMO)	No data
Seton Health Plan (Austin and Waco areas)	No data	AUSTN: Seton Health Plan
UnitedHealthCare of Texas (Austin, San Antonio, and Waco areas)	United HealthCare of Texas, Inc. - Central Texas	AUSTN: UnitedHealthcare of Texas; SANAN: UnitedHealthcare of Texas
UnitedHealthcare of Texas (Dallas-Ft. Worth area)	UnitedHealthcare of Texas, Inc. - Dallas	DALLA: UnitedHealthcare of Texas
UnitedHealthcare of Texas (Southeastern and southern Texas)	United HealthCare of Texas, Inc. - Houston	HOUST: UnitedHealthcare of Texas
Valley Baptist Health Plan (HMO) (Harlingen area)	Valley Baptist Health Plan, Inc. (HMO)	No data

Utah

Plan		
Altius Health Plans (Wasatch Front area)	Altius Health Plans	SALTL: Altius Health Plans
CIGNA HealthCare (Wasatch Front area)	CIGNA HealthCare	SALTL: CIGNA HealthCare of Utah
Intermountain Health Care (Most of Utah)	IHC	SALTL: IHC Care
Regence BlueCross BlueShield of UT/ HealthWise (All or most of UT)	RBCBSU	SALTL: HealthWise
SelectMed (Most of Utah)	No data	SALTL: SelectMed
UnitedHealthcare of Utah (Northern Utah)	UnitedHealthcare	SALTL: UnitedHealthcare of Utah
University of Utah Health Network (Wasatch Front area)	UUHN	No data

Vermont

Plan		
BlueCross BlueShield of Vermont (POS) (All of Vermont)	Blue Cross and Blue Shield of Vermont (POS)	No data
Harvard Pilgrim Health Care of New England (So. and eastern VT)	Harvard Pilgrim Health Care of New England (NH/VT)	No data
HMO New England (All or most of Vermont)	No data	FAIRF: HMO New England; HARTF: HMO New England
MVP Health Care (HMO) (All of Vermont)	MVP Health Plan (HMO)	No data
The Vermont Health Plan (All of VT)	The Vermont Health Plan	No data

Virginia

Plan		
Aetna U.S. Healthcare (Northern Virginia)	Aetna U.S. Healthcare Inc. - Maryland, DC and Virginia	WASDC: Aetna U.S. Healthcare; BALTI: Aetna U.S. Healthcare
Capital Care/CareFirst (Northern Virginia)	Capital Care, Inc.	WASDC: CapitalCare; BALTI: CareFirst BlueCross BlueShield
CIGNA HealthCare Mid-Atlantic (Northern Virginia)	CIGNA HealthCare Mid-Atlantic, Inc.	WASDC: CIGNA HealthCare Mid-Atlantic; BALTI: CIGNA HealthCare Mid-Atlantic
CIGNA HealthCare of Virginia (Most of VA)	CIGNA HealthCare of Virginia	No data
HealthKeepers (Most of Virginia)	HealthKeepers, Inc.	WASDC: Healthkeepers
John Deere Health Plan (HMO) (Southwestern Virginia)	John Deere Health Care, Inc. (HMO)	No data
Kaiser Foundation HP Mid-Atlantic States (HMO) (Northern VA)	Kaiser Foundation Health Plan of the Mid-Atlantic States, Inc. (HMO)	WASDC: Kaiser Foundation Health Plan; BALTI: Kaiser Foundation Health Plan
M.D. IPA (Most of Virginia)	MD - Individual Practice Association, Inc.	WASDC: M.D. IPA; BALTI: M.D. IPA; NORFO: M.D. IPA
Optima Health Plan (HMO) (Southeastern Virginia)	Optima Health Plan (HMO)	NORFO: OPTIMA Health Plan
Optima Health Plan (POS) (Southeastern Virginia)	Optima Health Insurance Company (POS)	NORFO: OPTIMA Health Plan
Optimum Choice (All or most of Virginia)	Optimum Choice, Inc.	WASDC: Optimum Choice; BALTI: Optimum Choice; NORFO: Optimum Choice
PARTNERS Nat'l HP of NC (Blacksburg, Danville, Lynch., Roanoke)	PARTNERS National Health Plan of North Carolina	CHARL: PARTNERS Nat'l HPs of NC; WSALM: PARTNERS Health Plans; TRIAN: PARTNERS Health Plans
Peninsula Health Care (All or most of Virginia)	Peninsula Health Care, Inc.	No data
Priority Health Care (Most of Virginia)	Priority Health Care, Inc.	WASDC: Priority Health Care; NORFO: Priority Health Care
Southern Hlth Svcs (Danville, Fredericksburg, Rich., Roanoke)	Southern Health Services, Inc.	No data
UnitedHealthcare of the Mid-Atlantic (HMO) (Northern Virginia)	United Healthcare of the Mid-Atlantic (HMO)	WASDC: UnitedHealthcare Mid-Atlantic; BALTI: UnitedHealthcare Mid-Atlantic

Washington

Plan		
Aetna U.S. Healthcare (Puget Sound area)	Aetna U.S. Healthcare, Inc. - Washington	SEATT: Aetna U.S. Healthcare
Group Health Cooperative (HMO) (Most of Washington)	Group Health Cooperative of Puget Sound (HMO)	SEATT: Group Health Cooperative
Group Health Options (Most of WA)	Group Health Options, Inc.	No data
Group Health Options (POS) (Most of WA)	Group Health Options, Inc. (POS)	No data
Health Net Health Plan of Oregon (Southeastern Washington)	No data	PORTL: Health Net Health Plan of Oregon
Kaiser Permanente Northwest (HMO) (Southwestern Washington)	Kaiser Foundation Health Plan of the Northwest, Inc. (HMO)	PORTL: Kaiser Permanente Northwest
KPS Health Plans (HMO) (Puget Sound)	Kitsap Physicians Service (HMO)	No data
PacifiCare of Oregon (HMO) (Southwestern Washington)	PacifiCare of Oregon, Inc. (HMO)	PORTL: PacifiCare of Oregon
PacifiCare of WA (HMO) (Puget Sound area and most of western WA)	PacifiCare of Washington, Inc. (HMO)	No data
Premera Blue Cross (All or most of WA)	Premera Blue Cross	SEATT: Permera HealthPlus
Providence Health Plans (Southwestern Washington)	Providence Health Plans - Oregon	PORTL: Providence Health Plan
Regence HMO Oregon (Southwestern WA)	Regence HMO Oregon	PORTL: RegenceHMO (BCBS of Oregon)
RegenceCare (Seattle area)	No data	SEATT: RegenceCare

West Virginia

Plan		
CIGNA HealthCare Mid-Atlantic (Beckley and Morgan counties)	CIGNA HealthCare Mid-Atlantic, Inc.	WASDC: CIGNA HealthCare Mid-Atlantic; BALTI: CIGNA HealthCare Mid-Atlantic
The Health Plan of the Upper Ohio Valley (HMO) (No.-central/NW WV)	The Health Plan of the Upper Ohio Valley, Inc. (HMO)	No data
HealthAmerica (HMO) (Northern West Virginia)	HealthAmerica Pennsylvania, Inc. (HMO)	PITTS: HealthAmerica of Pennsylvania
HealthAmerica (POS) (Northern WV)	HealthAmerica Pennsylvania, Inc. (POS)	PITTS: HealthAmerica of Pennsylvania
Optimum Choice (All or most of West Virginia)	Optimum Choice, Inc.	WASDC: Optimum Choice; BALTI: Optimum Choice; NORFO: Optimum Choice

Wisconsin

Plan		
CompcareBlue (All or most of Wisconsin)	Compcare Health Services Insurance Corporation	MILWA: CompcareBlue
Dean Health Plan (HMO) (Southern WI)	Dean Health Plan, Inc. (HMO)	No data
Group Health Cooperative of Eau Claire (HMO) (Eau Claire area)	Group Health Cooperative of Eau Claire (HMO)	No data
Group Health Cooperative of South Central WI (HMO) (Madison area)	Group Health Cooperative of South Central Wisconsin (HMO)	No data
Gunderson Lutheran Health Plan (HMO) (Southwestern Wisconsin)	Gunderson Lutheran Health Plan, Inc (HMO)	No data
HMO Illinois/BlueAdvantage (HMO) (Kenosha County)	HMO Illinois and Blue Advantage HMO (HMO)	CHICA: HMO Illinois
Humana Wisconsin (HMO) (Southeastern Wisconsin)	Humana Wisconsin Health Organization Insurance Corporation (HMO)	MILWA: Humana Wisconsin
Medica (Western Wisconsin)	Medica Health Plans	TWINC: Medica
Medical Associates Health Plans (Southwestern Wisconsin)	Medical Associates Health Plan, Inc. dba Medical Associates Health Plans	No data
Network Health Plan of Wisconsin (HMO) (Southeastern Wisconsin)	Network Health Plan of Wisconsin, Inc. (HMO)	No data
Physicians Plus (Southern Wisconsin)	Physicians Plus Insurance Corporation	No data
Security Health Plan (HMO) (Northern, western, and central Wisconsin)	Security Health Plan (HMO)	No data
Touchpoint Health Plan (HMO) (Northeastern Wisconsin)	Touchpoint Health Plan (HMO)	No data
Touchpoint Health Plan (POS) (Northeastern Wisconsin)	Touchpoint Health Plan (POS)	No data
UnitedHealthcare of Wisconsin (Southeastern Wisconsin)	UnitedHealthcare of Wisconsin	MILWA: UnitedHealthcare of Wisconsin
Unity Health Plans (Southwestern and south-central Wisconsin)	Unity Health Plans Insurance Corporation	No data
Valley Health Plan (Western Wisconsin)	Valley Health Plan	No data

Wyoming

Plan		
Intermountain Health Care (Parts of Western Wyoming)	IHC	SALTL: IHC Care

Key to Physicians Survey Region Codes and Counties Surveyed

ATLAN — Atlanta Area (including Cherokee, Clayton, Cobb, DeKalb, Douglas, Fayette, Fulton, Gwinnett, Henry, and Rockdale counties)

AUSTN — Austin Area (including Travis County)

BALTI — Baltimore Area (including Baltimore City and Baltimore County)

BOSTN — Boston Area (including Bristol, Essex, Middlesex, Norfolk, Plymouth, and Suffolk counties)

BUFFA — Buffalo Area (including Erie County)

CHARL — Charlotte Area (including Mecklenburg County)

CHICA — Chicago Area (including Cook, Du Page, Kane, Kendall, Lake, McHenry, and Will counties)

CINCI — Cincinnati Area (including Hamilton County)

CLEVE — Cleveland Area (including Cuyahoga County)

DALLA — Dallas-Ft. Worth Area (including Dallas and Tarrant counties)

COLUM — Columbus Area (including Franklin County)

DENVR — Denver Area (including Adams, Arapahoe, Denver, and Jefferson counties)

DETRO — Greater Detroit Area (including Macomb, Oakland, Washtenaw, and Wayne counties)

FAIRF — Fairfield and New Haven Counties Area

FTMEY — Charlotte, Collier, and Lee Counties Area

HARTF — Hartford Area (including Hartford County)

HOUST — Houston Area (including Harris County)

INDIAN — Indianapolis Area (including Marion County)

JERSE — Northern and Central New Jersey (including Bergen, Essex, Hudson, Hunterdon, Middlesex, Monmouth, Morris, Passaic, Somerset, Sussex, Union, and Warren counties)

KCITY — Kansas City Area (including Johnson and Wyandotte counties in Kansas and Jackson County, Missouri)

LOSAN — Los Angeles and Orange Counties Area

MILWA — Milwaukee Area (including Milwaukee County)

NASHV — Nashville Area (including Davidson County)

NEWOR — New Orleans Area (including Orleans Parrish)

NORFO — Norfolk Area (including the city of Norfolk)

NYORK — New York City, Long Island, and Westchester County

ORLAN — Brevard, Orange, Seminole, and Volusia Counties Area

PHILA — Greater Philadelphia Area (including Bucks, Chester, Delaware, Montgomery, and Philadelphia counties in Pennsylvania; Burlington, Camden, and Gloucester counties in New Jersey; and New Castle County, Delaware)

PHOEN — Phoenix Area (including Maricopa County)

PITTS — Pittsburgh Area (including Allegheny County)

PORTL — Portland Area (including Clackamas, Multnomah, and Washington counties)

RHODE — Rhode Island (including all of Rhode Island)

RIVER — Riverside and San Bernardino Counties Area

ROCHE — Rochester Area (including Monroe County)

SACRA — Sacramento Area (including Sacramento County)

SALTL — Salt Lake City Area (including Salt Lake County)

SANAN — San Antonio Area (including Bexar County)

SDIEG — San Diego Area (including San Diego County)

SEATT — Seattle Area (including King, Kitsap, Pierce, and Snohomish counties)

SFRAN — San Francisco Bay Area (including Alameda, Contra Costa, Marin, Napa, San Francisco, Santa Clara, Solano, and Sonoma counties)

SOFLA — South Florida (including Broward, Miami-Dade, Monroe, and Palm Beach counties)

STLOU — St. Louis Area (including St. Louis City and St. Louis County)

TAMPA — Hillsborough, Manatee, Pinellas, Polk, and Sarasota Counties Area

TRIAN — Triangle Area (including Durham, Orange, and Wake counties)

TWINC — Twin Cities Area (including Anoka, Carver, Dakota, Hennepin, Ramsey, Scott, Washington, and Wright counties)

VEGAS — Las Vegas Area (including Clark County)

WASHI — Washington, DC, Area (including the District of Columbia; Anne Arundel, Howard, Montgomery, and Prince George's counties in Maryland; and Alexandria, Arlington County, Fairfax County, Loudoun County, and Prince William County in Virginia)

WSALM — Forsyth and Guilford Counties Area

Appendix B

State Insurance Counseling Programs

Alabama
1-800-243-5463 or
334-242-5743

Alaska
1-800-478-6065 or
907-269-3680

Arizona
1-800-432-4040 or
602-542-6595

Arkansas
1-800-224-6330 or
501-371-2782

California
1-800-434-0222

Colorado
1-888-696-7213 or
303-899-5151

Connecticut
1-800-994-9422 or
860-424-5245

Delaware
1-800-336-9500 or
302-739-6266

District of Columbia
202-739-0668

Florida
1-800-963-5337 or
850-414-2060

Georgia
1-800-669-8387 or
404-657-5334

Hawaii
1-888-875-9229 or
808-586-7299

Idaho
1-800-247-4422 or
208-334-4350

Illinois
1-800-548-9034 or
217-785-9021

Indiana
1-800-452-4800 or
317-233-3475

Iowa
1-800-351-4664 or
515-281-6867

Kansas
1-800-860-5260 or
316-337-7386

Kentucky
1-877-293-7447

Louisiana
1-800-259-5301 or
225-342-5301

Maine
1-800-750-5353 or
207-623-1797

Maryland
1-800-243-3425 or
410-767-1100

Massachusetts
1-800-882-2003

Michigan
1-800-803-7174 or
517-886-0899

Minnesota
1-800-333-2433

Mississippi
1-800-948-3090 or
601-359-4929

Missouri
1-800-390-3330

Montana
1-800-332-2272 or
406-444-4077

Nebraska
1-800-234-7119 or
402-471-2201

Nevada
1-800-307-4444 or
702-486-3478

New Hampshire
1-800-852-3388 or
603-225-9000

New Jersey
1-800-792-8820 or
609-943-3437

New Mexico
1-800-432-2080 or
505-827-7640

New York
1-800-333-4114 or
212-869-3850

North Carolina
1-800-443-9354 or
919-733-0111

North Dakota
1-800-247-0560 or
701-328-2440

Ohio
800-686-1578 or
614-644-3458

Oklahoma
1-800-763-2828 or
405-521-6628

Oregon
1-800-722-4134 or
503-947-7984

Pennsylvania
1-800-783-7067 or
570-347-5616

Puerto Rico
1-877-725-4300 or
787-721-8590

Rhode Island
401-222-2880

South Carolina
1-800-868-9095 or
803-898-2850

South Dakota
1-800-822-8804 or
605-773-3656

Tennessee
1-877-801-0044 or
615-242-0438

Texas
1-800-252-9240 or
512-424-6840

Utah
1-800-541-7735 or
801-538-3910

Vermont
1-800-642-5119 or
802-748-5182

Virginia
1-800-552-3402 or
804-662-9333

Washington
1-800-397-4422 or
360-664-3154

West Virginia
1-877-987-4463 or
304-558-3317

Wisconsin
1-800-242-1060 or
608-267-3298

Wyoming
1-800-856-4398 or
307-856-6880

Appendix C

State Health Insurance Regulators

Alabama
Department of Insurance
P.O. Box 303351
Montgomery, AL 36130-3351
334-241-4141

Alaska
Division of Insurance
Department of Commerce and
  Economic Development
3601 C Street, Suite 1324
Anchorage, AK 99503
907-465-4607

Arizona
Department of Insurance
2910 N. 44th Street, Suite 210
Phoenix, AZ 85018-7256
602-912-8456

Arkansas
Department of Insurance
1200 W. 3rd Street
Little Rock, AR 72201-1904
501-371-2766

California
Department of Insurance
Consumer Communications
  Bureau
300 S. Spring Street, South Tower
Los Angeles, CA 90013
1-800-927-4357 or
  213-897-8921

Colorado
Division of Insurance
1560 Broadway, Suite 850
Denver, CO 80202
303-894-7499

Connecticut
Department of Insurance
P.O. Box 816
Hartford, CT 06142-0816
860-297-3812

Delaware
Department of Insurance
Rodney Building
841 Silver Lake Boulevard
Dover, DE 19904
302-739-4251

District of Columbia
Department of Insurance and
  Securities Regulation
810 First Street, N.E., Suite 701
Washington, DC 20002
202-442-7758

Florida
Department of Insurance
200 E. Gaines Street
Larson Building
Tallahassee, FL 32399-0321
850-413-5110

Georgia
Department of Insurance
2 Martin Luther King, Jr. Drive
Floyd Memorial Building
716 West Tower
Atlanta, GA 30334
404-656-2085

Hawaii
Insurance Division
Department of Commerce and
  Consumer Affairs
250 S. King Street, 5th Floor
Honolulu, HI 96813
808-586-2809

Idaho
Department of Insurance
700 W. State Street, 3rd Floor
Boise, ID 83720-0043
208-334-4300

Illinois
Office of Consumer Health
  Insurance
Department of Insurance
320 W. Washington Street, 4th Fl.
Springfield, IL 62767
1-877-527-9431

Indiana
Department of Insurance
311 W. Washington Street
Indianapolis, IN 46204-2787
317-232-5695

Iowa
Division of Insurance
330 E. Maple Street
Des Moines, IA 50319
515-281-6836

Kansas
Department of Insurance
420 S.W. 9th Street
Topeka, KS 66612-1678
785-296-7807

Kentucky
Department of Insurance
P.O. Box 517
Frankfort, KY 40602-0517
502-564-6029

Louisiana
Office of Health
Quality Management Division
P.O. Box 94214
Baton Rouge, LA 70804-9214
225-219-4770

Maine
Bureau of Insurance
Department of Professional and
  Financial Regulation
State Office Building, Station 34
Augusta, ME 04333-0034
207-624-8428

Maryland
Insurance Administration
525 St. Paul Place
Baltimore, MD 21202-2272
410-468-2201

Massachusetts
Division of Insurance
One South Station, 5th Floor
Boston, MA 02110
617-521-7364

Michigan
Insurance Division
Office of Financial and Insurance
  Services
611 W. Ottawa Street, 2nd Floor
Lansing, MI 48933-1020
517-373-2984

Minnesota
Department of Commerce
85 7th Place E., Suite 500
St. Paul, MN 55101-2198
651-296-8949

Mississippi
Insurance Department
1804 Walter Sillers Building
P.O. Box 79
Jackson, MS 39205
601-359-2453

Missouri
Department of Insurance
P.O. Box 690
Jefferson City, MO 65102-0690
573-751-4363

Montana
Department of Insurance
840 Helena Avenue
Helena, MT 59601
406-444-4613

Nebraska
Department of Insurance
Terminal Building, Suite 400
941 'O' Street
Lincoln, NE 68508
402-471-2850

Nevada
Division of Insurance
788 Fairview Drive, Suite 300
Carson City, NV 89701-5491
775-687-4270

New Hampshire
Department of Insurance
56 Old Suncook Road
Concord, NH 03301
603-271-2261

New Jersey
Department of Banking and
    Insurance
P.O. Box 325
Trenton, NJ 08625
609-984-3602

New Mexico
Department of Insurance
P.O. Drawer 1269
Santa Fe, NM 87504-1269
505-827-4625

New York
Consumer Services Bureau
Insurance Department
Agency Building One
Empire State Plaza
Albany, NY 12257
1-800-342-3736 or
    518-474-6600

North Carolina
Department of Insurance
P.O. Box 26387
Raleigh, NC 27611
919-733-5060

North Dakota
Department of Insurance
600 E. Boulevard Avenue
Bismarck, ND 58505-0320
701-328-2489

Ohio
Department of Insurance
2100 Stella Court
Columbus, OH 43215-1067
614-644-2658

Oklahoma
Department of Insurance
2401 N.W. 23rd Street, Suite 28
Oklahoma City, OK 73107
405-521-3541

Oregon
Division of Insurance
Department of Consumer and
    Business Services
350 Winter Street N.E.
Salem, OR 97301-3883
503-947-7205

Pennsylvania
Insurance Department
1321 Strawberry Square
Harrisburg, PA 17120
717-787-0684

Puerto Rico
Department of Insurance
P.O. Box 8330
San Juan, PR 09910
787-722-8686

Rhode Island
Insurance Division
Department of Business
    Regulation
233 Richmond Street, Suite 233
Providence, RI 02903-4233
401-222-2223

South Carolina
Department of Insurance
P.O. Box 100105
Columbia, SC 29202-3105
803-737-6165

South Dakota
Division of Insurance
Department of Commerce and
    Regulation
118 W. Capitol Avenue
Pierre, SD 57501-2000
605-773-3563

Tennessee
Department of Commerce and
    Insurance
Volunteer Plaza
500 James Robertson Parkway
Nashville, TN 37243-0574
615-741-2199

Texas
Department of Insurance
333 Guadalupe Street
P.O. Box 149104
Austin, TX 78714-9104
512-305-6788

Utah
Department of Insurance
3110 State Office Building
Salt Lake City, UT 84114-1201
801-538-9656

Vermont
Consumer Services
Division of Health Care
    Administration
Department of Banking,
    Insurance, and Securities
89 Main Street, Drawer 20
Montpelier, VT 05620-3601
1-800-631-7788 or
    802-828-2900

Virginia
Bureau of Insurance
State Corporation Commission
P.O. Box 1157
Richmond, VA 23218
804-371-9074

Washington
Office of the Insurance
    Commissioner
14th Avenue & Water Streets
P.O. Box 40256
Olympia, WA 98504-0256
360-753-3613

West Virginia
Department of Insurance
P.O. Box 50540
Charleston, WV 25305-0540
304-558-0401

Wisconsin
Office of the Insurance
    Commissioner
P.O. Box 7873
Madison, WI 53707
608-266-7726

Wyoming
Department of Insurance
Herschler Building
122 W. 25th Street, 3rd East
Cheyenne, WY 82002-0440
307-777-6807

change and, 107; meetings for, 69; organization of, 68; prioritizing problems using, 120; relationship map in, 80–83; results of, 72; revising process descriptions in, 95; tools for, 70–72; work flow over the physical space in, 87–90

Technical process design, 133–148; challenging assumptions and mapping alternative work flows in, 137–142; designing new work flow in, 143–145; finalizing technical design in, 146–148; human systems design and, 170; meetings for, 135; organization of, 134; purpose of, 133; results of, 135

Technical processes: designing a work system and, 28; finding problems with, 96–100; initiation and scoping and, 31; need for design due to conditions in, 6; as one part of system, 6, 13, 15; performance analysis of, 8, 13

Tools: environmental analysis with, 58; human systems analysis with, 104–105; technical processes analysis with, 70–72. *See also specific tools*

Training: attempting to resolve problems through, 3, 8, 31, 150; building and training skills through, 17; determining requirements and levels of satisfaction and, 60; human systems design and, 173–175

Tryout assessment flowchart, 193

V

Value added, and design improvements, 9

Values and norms, in human structure and support systems, 17, 25, 101, 150

Van Gundy, A. B., 37

Variance analysis worksheet, 235; analyzing structures and human resource systems with, 112; case study of, 219; departure from specifications shown on, 72; finding problems with current technical processes using, 100; mapping alternative work flows with, 137; role of managers in new system and, 154

W

Westgaard, O., 58

Work flow: analysis of technical processes and, 25; case study of new process, 212–213, 222–223; defining desired outcomes and, 36; designing, 143–145; fragmentation of, 3–6; identifying, 87–90; mapping alternative, 137–142; purpose of, 87; requirements for starting, 87; samples of, 88–90; steps and specifics for, 87; technical process analysis and, 15, 67, 133; tools for analyzing, 70; when to use, 87

Work-flow chart, 70; creating a relationship map with, 81; examples of, 78–79, 141–142; finding problems with current technical process using, 97–98; mapping alternative work flows with, 137

Work group: analyzing the existing system and, 26; analyzing structures and human resource systems and, 112; human systems design and principles of, 158, 159; relationship map of, 80–83

Work group design, 10; appearance of, 12; different environments needing different approaches to, 14; results of, 13; training in, 60

Work process: assumptions about, 140; comparison of group boundaries to, 104; definition of, 47; good design and appearance of, 11; setting goals for the design and, 126, 127

Worksheets: business environment matrix, 64; cycle time, 70, 91, 92, 93–94, 233–234; desired process outcomes, 77, 200–203; process parameters, 215–217; responsibility development, 162; variance analysis, 72, 100, 112, 154, 235

Work space map, 70